Ovulation Stimulation with Gonadotropins

Jean-Claude Emperaire

Ovulation Stimulation with Gonadotropins

Foreword by Bruno Lunenfeld

Springer

Jean-Claude Emperaire
Bordeaux
France

This work is a translation from the book: Emperaire J.C., Pratique de la stimulation ovulatoire par les gonadotrophines, Springer-Verlag France, ISBN: 978-2-8178-0397-5, 2013

ISBN 978-3-319-18653-5 ISBN 978-3-319-18654-2 (eBook)
DOI 10.1007/978-3-319-18654-2

Library of Congress Control Number: 2015947362

Springer Cham Heidelberg New York Dordrecht London

Printed on acid-free paper

Springer International Publishing AG Switzerland is part of Springer Science+Business Media (www.springer.com)

To my beloved wife Cosette and sons
Pierre and Julien

Foreword

Gonadotropin therapy is so central to infertility treatment that it is easy to overlook the considerable discovery and research that preceded our understanding of the reproductive process, diagnostic procedures, treatment protocols, and the production of the effective and safe therapeutic agents available today.

The history underpinning this development spans over 300 years and provides a splendid example of how basic animal experimentation and technological advances have progressed to clinical application.

Following the discovery of germ cells in 1677, and the realization that fertilization involved the merging of two cell nuclei, one from the egg and one from sperm, in 1870, it took another 40 years to discover the interplay between the hypothalamus, pituitary, and gonads in 1910.

The gonadotropins were discovered in 1927. Gonadotropins, such as pregnant mare serum gonadotropin (PMSG), were first introduced for ovarian stimulation in 1930. However, the use of PMSG led to antibody formation and had to be withdrawn. Following our discovery that urinary menopausal gonadotropins (HMG) could stimulate gonadal function in 1953, and the delivery of the first child by our group in 1961, the path opened to controlled ovarian stimulation. Human pituitary gonadotropins extracted from pituitaries of cadavers (HPG) produced good results, but its use came to an end in the late 1980s when it was linked to the development of Creutzfeldt-Jakob disease.

With the availability of HMG, clomiphene citrate, ergot derivatives, GnRH agonists and antagonists, as well as metformin, algorithms were developed and have been used successfully to treat infertility for the past four decades.

Following Heape's first rabbit embryo transfers in 1880, Pincus' attempts at IVF in rabbits in 1934, Menkin and Rock's in vitro fertilization of human eggs in 1944, and Chang's rabbit birth following IVF, the first human IVF baby was born from a natural cycle in 1978.

Following the first IVF baby born after gonadotropin stimulation in 1981, IVF procedures became standard practice for the management of tubal factor infertility and increased the demand of gonadotropins significantly. The demand was further increased after donor embryo and donor egg transfer technology permitted treating women with ovarian failure, and intracytoplasmic injection of a single spermatozoon into an oocyte opened the way to treat male infertility.

The main agents for controlled ovarian stimulation for IVF were gonadotropins and GnRH analogues, and it soon became evident that there would never be a sufficient urine supply to cover the increasing world demand for gonadotropins.

Recombinant DNA technology now allows the production of pharmacologically active pure FSH, LH, and hCG preparations in unlimited quantities, minimizing any potential risk of disease transmission via biological contamination. The introduction of recombinant gonadotropins with more than 99 % purity gradually replaced HMG preparations worldwide.

With batch to batch consistency of gonadotropin preparations, methods could be developed to predict and select the correct dose and the optimal protocol for each patient. In 2012 it was calculated that assisted reproductive technology with the use of gonadotropins for ovulation induction has helped couples deliver more than 12 million children: 7 million after ovulation induction or intrauterine insemination and another 5 million through in vitro fertilization.

However, examination of worldwide results reveals still wide variations in live birth rates. This situation could be changed if women would seek treatment before the age of 35, if clinicians would use optimal protocols to diagnose and manage their patients, and if embryologists would use the best tools to select the best embryo. All this we can learn from this small but precise volume.

As a highly experienced and well-recognized specialist, Dr. Jean-Claude Emperaire describes the correct use of these protocols in a very didactic and scientific manner in this book. This volume will help clinicians to a better understanding of the physiology of reproduction, the therapeutic agents they use, and the management of patients with subfertility and infertility to obtain the best possible, most cost-effective results.

Bruno Lunenfeld, MD, PhD, FRCOG, FACOG (Hon)
Professor Emeritus, Faculty of Life Sciences, Bar-Ilan University, Israel
General Secretary, Asian Pacific Initiative on Reproductive Endocrinology

Preface

Most infertile couples will eventually attempt procedures to stimulate ovulation, whether as first-line therapy or for assisted conception. Although the process of controlled ovarian hyperstimulation (COH) for in vitro fertilization (IVF) purposes generally requires the skilled experience of a specialist, a mono- or pauci-follicular stimulation can and should be guided by a patient's own gynecologist with whom she has a longer trusting relationship. To be sure, every stimulation cycle contains some risk for ovarian hyperstimulation and/or a multiple pregnancy, and these possibilities do create a degree of apprehension among clinicians who may be considering the procedure. In addition, as happens with most therapies that promise a significant benefit, ovulation protocols can be fraught with so many unwieldy variations and details that many clinicians simply decline to become involved. Stimulation of ovulation is in fact a simple treatment and quite uncomplicated for most patients. Although there is not yet a particular accreditation or certification for clinicians who aspire to conduct classic ovulation stimulations, or even one governing the use of COH protocols, it is nevertheless possible to assure a low-risk sequence of events to one's patients.

So then, how does one learn to stimulate ovulation effectively? Usually it has been self-taught owing to inaccessibility of an experienced mentor. But the process includes numerous decisions and choices regarding patient evaluation, gonadotropin preparations, posology, protocols, duration of treatments, and when and how to trigger ovulation. Proper, safe stimulation requires an insightful anticipation of ovarian reactions. A clinician lacking experience to distinguish the unexpected from the unpredictable can easily lose confidence and focus when confronted by an unforeseen ovarian response. As one's practice moves to firmer ground, and fears of unknown areas dissipate, it becomes easier to learn and progress from each cycle failure without continually questioning whether a different strategy might have yielded a better outcome.

Evidence-based consensus is generally lacking with regard to ovulation stimulation, and, to some extent, there seem to be as many ways to manage certain situations as there are practitioners in the field, even among those within the same clinic team. Nevertheless, many basic rules do in fact exist, even as some might be interpreted by each clinician in accordance with personal views.

Thus it becomes all the more important to listen to the voices of experience. This handbook draws upon more than 30,000 classic and IVF stimulation cycles conducted over the past 40 years by the same clinician and particularly from the most recent thousand cycles that resulted in a clinical pregnancy. Nonetheless, it should be quickly apparent to the reader that protocols and strategies are not described here in exclusive terms. Indeed, all we are claiming is that these approaches have resulted in pregnancies. Similar outcomes might have been obtained with alternative approaches. The book is likewise not intended to take on numerous ethical or societal questions concerning the legitimacy of ovulation stimulation.

The sole ambition of this handbook is to allow each clinician who considers entrance into the field of ovarian stimulation to gain his/her own experience using these basic findings as a starting point while respecting the unique qualities of each patient and maintaining one's own judgment in the face of continued pronouncements of the statistically sure or medically correct.

Because most of the book's content is drawn on generally accepted knowledge, and from the author's own practice experiences, the bibliography has been kept to a minimum.

The author wishes to acknowledge the essential contributions to this English translation by Professor J. Charles Eldridge of the Wake Forest University School of Medicine in North Carolina. Dr. Eldridge has been a valued colleague and friend since our time of collaborative study in the Department of Endocrinology (Pr. R.B. Greenblatt) at the Medical College of Georgia and the Faculté de Médecine, Université de Bordeaux. His bilingual expertise and scholarship in reproductive endocrinology were invaluable for this version. Bravo, mon vieux, et mille merci.

Jean-Claude Emperaire, M.D.
Bordeaux, France

Abbreviations

AMH	Anti-Mullerian hormone
CD	Cycle day
CHO	Chinese hamster ovary
CNS	Central nervous system
COH	Controlled ovarian hyperstimulation
CTP	Carboxyl terminal peptide
FSH	Follicle-stimulating hormone
FSH-r	FSH receptor
GnRH	Gonadotropin-releasing hormone
GPR	G protein-coupled receptor
hCG	Human chorionic gonadotropin
HMG	Human menopausal gonadotropins
HMG-HP	HMG highly purified
HPG	Human pituitary gonadotropins
IRP	International reference preparation
IVF	In vitro fertilization
LH	Luteinizing hormone
LH-r	LH receptor
LUF	Luteinized unruptured follicle
MW	Molecular weight
OHSS	Ovarian hyperstimulation syndrome
PCOD	Polycystic ovarian disease
PMSG	Pregnant mare serum gonadotropins
POR	Poor ovarian response
rFSH	Recombinant FSH
r-hCG	Recombinant hCG
rLH	Recombinant LH
SNP	Single nuclear polymorphism
uFSH	Urinary FSH
u-hCG	Urinary hCG
uLH	Urinary LH
VEGF	Vascular endothelial growth factor

Contents

Historical Perspective: An Evolution of Ideas

1

Contemplating the evolution of the varied clinical uses of pituitary gonadotropic hormones reveals a number of interesting assumptions, and absence of assumptions, that have led us to present-day practices. While strategies for stimulating ovulation have steadily improved over the past 50 years, the basic principles governing clinical practice, e.g., indications for use, protocol design, and precautionary limits and hazards, were almost completely defined during the first decade of use. One exception to this might be the more recent protocol modifications adopted to stimulate ovulation for the purpose of in vitro fertilization (IVF).

To be sure, some protocol modifications represent true progress, namely the use of progressive "step-up" dosing in certain anovulatory situations, and also the recent success with patient self-administration. On the other hand, other modern developments, such as the arrival of a recombinant synthetic product, that importantly diversifies the supply source, have brought little effective change to either the fundamental principles of gonadotropin use or indeed to the success of ovulation stimulation.

Furthermore, some of the allegedly modern advances in protocols can be traced back to earlier concepts that were simply "forgotten" for a time. Examples include the concept of an "FSH threshold," essentially proposed by Brown in 1978 [1], the "FSH window," explored by Lunenfeld as early as 1961 [2], and the work of Donini testing preparations of varying FSH/LH ratios in 1968 [3]. In addition, the practice of "coasting" therapy as a way to lessen the risk of ovarian hyperstimulation and multiple pregnancies was being used by Delafontaine in 1978 even before the critical advance of ultrasound imaging [4].

1.1 Gonadotropins

Through the years, gonadotropin preparations for clinical use have been derived from four successive sources; the two most recent remain in use [5].

J.-C. Emperaire, *Ovulation Stimulation with Gonadotropins*,
DOI 10.1007/978-3-319-18654-2_1

1.1.1 Pregnant Mare's Serum Gonadotropins (PMSG)

Preparations of PMSG first appeared in 1937 and successful clinical use to stimulate ovarian follicular growth in patients was achieved as early as 1941. However, a rapidly-developing immune response was soon recognized, that rendered patients insensitive to further treatment after only a few trials. As a result clinical uses of this product were soon abandoned.

1.1.2 Human Pituitary Gonadotropins (HPG)

Following the clinical failure of PMSG, ovulation stimulation was attempted with an extract of human pituitary tissue. First applied in 1958, the extracts achieved modest success and continued in use until 1988, when the cases of associated Creutzfeldt-Jakob disease became evident. Although clinical use of this preparation would have always been limited by a meager supply of source tissue, these pituitary extracts remain useful today as International Reference Preparations.

1.1.3 Human Menopausal Gonadotropins (HMG)

The ability to isolate and purify hormones from the urine of post-menopausal women ushered in the true era of gonadotropin use. Using a kaolin-acetone extraction method, Bruno Lunenfeld demonstrated as early as 1945 that it was possible to isolate and purify gonadotropins from menopausal urines. Injections of the extract into immature rats stimulated ovarian follicular growth and testicular spermatogenesis in the testis. Although the potential clinical value of these preparations was easy to predict, it remained impossible to patent this natural human product and thus difficult to convince pharmaceutical companies to engage a project that required massive urine collections, construction of an industrial-sized extraction technology, and development of the necessary safety precautions, based solely on hypotheses derived from animal experiments.

The true history of HMG development finally began in Rome in 1957 when Pietro Donini, a senior research scientist who had extracted HMG at the Instituto Farmacologico Serono, invited Professor Lunenfeld to visit and discuss with the institute's board the feasibility of mass producing HMG and initiating clinical trials. Initially the proposal was not well received, due to little enthusiasm to convert laboratories into commercial urinals. Fortunately, the Vatican had been holding a major share in the Instituto Farmacologico Serono since 1952, and Don Giulio Pacelli was their representative to the board. He also happened to be a nephew of the Pope and began to take an interest in the project. Professor Lunenfeld was asked to remain in Rome for continued discussions that led to a proposal that the homes of retired nuns could provide ample supplies of urine. The Serono board was convinced to undertake the project.

This offer proved to be very successful: by 1961 Lunenfeld was able to report the first newborn infants from ova stimulated by HMG injections [6], and by this time three collection centers, in Italy, Spain, and the Netherlands, were already operating with more than 600 donors. This same method of HMG production for direct ovarian stimulation continues in use to the present time.

For many years human menopausal gonadotropins remained the only direct ovarian stimulator, and the essentials of stimulation strategy were written through its use. Because the post-menopausal woman is hypogonadal and hypergonadotropic, FSH and LH appear at significant levels in urine. Only a very limited degree of hepatic and renal metabolism occurs, which allows retention of most biological properties.

FSH isoforms in urinary HMG are slightly more acidic, partly because its extremely elevated secretion in hypoestrogenic women contains more of the acidic isoforms, and partly because the acidic isoform population survives hepatic and renal metabolism better. LH content of HMG extracts is proportionately lower than FSH because post-menopausal women secrete more FSH than LH. In order to balance therapeutic concentration of the two hormones closer to equality, it was initially necessary to add pregnancy urine-extracted hCG, the only other hormone preparation available at that time with true LH-like activity. This supplementation was actually unidentified but was suspected for a long time by clinicians. It has only recently been acknowledged by pharmaceutical companies because radioimmunoassay technology has made it possible to distinguish pituitary LH from hCG. hCG supplementation of HMG preparations is no longer permitted and the pharmaceutical manufacturers now claim that a balanced ratio of FSH/LH is achieved by the presence of pituitary hCG that supposedly occurs naturally in post-menopausal urine.

Initially FSH potency varied substantially in the vials supplied by the pioneering manufacturers Serono (*Pergonal®*, later *Neopergonal®*) and Organon (*Humegon®*) that led to variable clinical responses as well. This was likely the result of using a wide variety of urine donors and extraction procedures, and also of using imprecise bioassays to establish international reference units (IU). Vials labeled as containing 75 IU each of FSH and LH could in fact range from 55 to 80 IU of either hormone. Clinicians often blamed these potency variations as the cause of irregular results from IVF procedures, although early embryology technology also brought a number of uncertainties.

Up through the 1980s, the preparations of hMG permitted a satisfactory cure for most dysovulatory or anovulatory patients, save those afflicted with polycystic ovarian disease (PCOD). Initially known as the Stein-Leventhal syndrome, PCOD is typified by excess body weight, anovulation, hyperandrogenism, and an excessive LH secretion that produces a lower serum FSH/LH ratio, along with a possible metabolic syndrome with an enhanced risk of Type II diabetes mellitus. Pathophysiology of this syndrome was believed to result from a relative shortfall of FSH secretion accompanied by LH excess, and it was initially proposed that treatment with pure FSH would restore successful ovulations.

Although this assumption was later shown to be incorrect, it did lend energy to resolving the purity problems of HMG, and a more purified FSH product (uFSH) appeared in 1988. Nevertheless, this preparation offered no therapeutic improvement. It took a return to the original principles of defining an FSH threshold, and the design of a slower "step-up" protocol, to restore normal ovulations in PCOD patients. It turned out that rates of both success and complications were quite the same, whether hMG or uFSH were used [7].

Development of a refined uFSH preparation became the last example of a progressive step initially sought by clinicians, and to which the manufacturers responded. In a considerable shift of roles, most all of the subsequent developments in gonadotropin preparations have been initiated by the pharmaceutical companies themselves. In the meantime, the market for gonadotropin preparations has been greatly expanded due to increased use for in vitro fertilization procedures. From a "craft" developed and practiced by a relatively small number of gynecologic specialists, the therapeutic approaches to infertility have blossomed into a substantial industry, and include a new set of philosophies and practices. This has resulted in significant conflicts between product design and marketing on the one hand, and uses of therapeutic agents and therapeutic goals on the other.

Coincidentally, marketing strategies put increased pressure on scientific and medical issues. It is important to keep in mind the recent episode of LH slander that occurred simultaneously with the arrival of uFSH. Although pituitary LH was long known as a valuable physiologic promoter of steroidogenesis in ovarian follicles and corpora lutea, the hormone became suddenly and repeatedly attacked during many congresses and symposia as a deleterious therapeutic agent, allegedly responsible for miscarriages, infertility, and other forms of reproductive failure. Although the campaign was disguised as honest scientific debate, it appears to have been little more than a scheme of adverse publicity to discredit hMG preparations. The fact that many clinicians were dragged in good faith into this marketing ploy clearly demonstrates the power that pharmaceutical companies have acquired in order to control initiatives in research and development. Through positions of influence conferred by sponsorship of professional conferences and clinician training programs, corporations continually tout the advantages of their new products. The LH example should cause clinicians to retain an open mind when confronted with these short-lived "truths" and assertions.

Although medical practice welcomed the arrival of purified urinary FSH (uFSH), and later highly purified urinary FSH (uFSH-HP), there remained a problem of supply. Thus the development of genetically synthesized recombinant FSH (rFSH), followed soon by rLH and r-hCG, now offers a valuable and potentially inexhaustible supply of these hormones. However, as typically befalls existing pharmaceuticals, the arrival of "something new" is accompanied by heavy publicity designed primarily to discredit the existing medications they seek to replace. This is regrettable because the urinary gonadotropin extracts were never clinically inadequate, and never deserved to fall from grace. They remain highly valuable FSH preparations.

1.1.4 Recombinant FSH (rFSH)

Once the genes coding for the two subunits of FSH were isolated, it was a simple task to transfect cDNA into appropriate cell lines. Two Chinese hamster ovary (CHO) cell lines, one containing two plasmids and the other one plasmid, are used to produce, respectively, follitropin alpha (*Gonal F*®) and follitropin beta (*Puregon*®). As a result, many challenges and problems of natural hormone extracts have been resolved through genetic engineering. The supply is now inexhaustible, batch-to-batch variation has been eliminated, and there is no contamination by foreign (urine) proteins. On the other hand, some of the more recent advances by pharmaceutical companies, namely defining FSH potency by mass rather than bioassay units, or releasing products with specific FSH/LH ratios such as 2/1, or developing longer-acting preparations, all appear to be targeted more toward postponement of patent expirations than to increasing interest among clinicians and their patients. An example of this so-called progress is the filling of FSH injection pens with an identified mass quantity (micrograms) of hormone rather than with international units, in an effort to suppress all batch-to-batch variation that does remain possible with bioassay measures. Such a sophistication is substantially dampened in daily clinical practice by the large fluctuations in ovarian response that occur from one treatment cycle to another in the same patient using the same FSH dosage.

In summary, advances in ovarian stimulation since the appearance of hMG may be summarized in two basic ways: (1) the use of "step-up" low doses and chronic low dose protocols, particularly for PCOD patients; (2) the ability of patients to self-administer the more stable synthetic product, thus permitting infertile couples to participate together in a more personalized therapeutic schedule.

One potential technological advance that has little likelihood of occurring is the availability of LH for triggering ovulation. Unfortunately, the presently-used hCG, whether as a urine extract or a recombinant product, is primarily responsible for ovarian hyperstimulation and multiple pregnancies. Despite a final wish by clinicians to be able to trigger ovulation with synthetic LH or an LH-like molecule, these advanced preparations seem unlikely to become available for that purpose, not because the means to produce it are lacking, but rather because there is little profit incentive to conduct the necessary research. Although manufacturers continue to assert their concern for patient safety, on this particular issue they will continue to do nothing.

1.2 Monitoring Ovarian Stimulation

During the many years when only hMG was available, the principal advance of methodology was the very critical ability to monitor responses to the stimulation: first by measures of follicular estrogen secretion, and then by morphologic criteria using reliable ultrasound imagery.

Initially, estimation of the ovarian response to gonadotropins was possible only through observation of clinically available estrogen target tissues, e.g., vaginal mucosa and the uterine cervix. Examination of target tissue responses such as the vaginal eosinophilic index, cervical mucus, and opening of the cervical external os, were unfortunately of little help, because of typically large variances between patients. Even within the same patient, a dose-response relationship could be imprecise, especially in cases when a maximal response was achieved at relatively low estrogen levels. Significantly improved assessment was not provided even when combined with other clinical observations, such as ovarian volume and sensitivity through vaginal examination. These difficulties explain much of the early occurrence of ovarian hyperstimulation syndrome that unfortunately ended on occasion with a patient's death.

1.2.1 Monitoring by Hormonal Measures

The first revolutionary advance toward improved monitoring used measures of ovarian estrogen production, initially estimated indirectly by quantifying urinary excretion of estrogen metabolites. Although long available, the usual assay typically required a lengthy turn-around time of up to 3 days. Assay protocols included a prolonged hydrolysis step followed by extraction of the phenolic steroids from urine, but this was of little use to a therapeutic situation where estrogen production could vary continually. Attempts at a more rapid hydrolysis with boiling NaOH proved even less useful because the estrogen analytes were partially degraded, and assay results were tempered.

Ruffié and Jayle deserve considerable credit for improving the steroid hydrolysis step in 1965, by increasing the concentration of a hydrolytic enzyme catalyst (obtained from snails) as well as the temperature of the reaction. Adopting a Kober-Ittrich spectro-fluorometric analysis of the extract yielded a good same-day result from urine specimens collected during the previous 24 h [8].

Availability of this "rapid" total estrogen assay began to diminish the importance of some imprecise clinical observations, save perhaps the evaluation of cervical mucus, and it produced a much better risk estimate for ovarian hyperstimulation. Because the optimal margin of safety was close to the normal preovulatory estrogen level of 30–100 μg/24 h, it became important to add a creatinine assay to assure that a complete 24 h sample had been collected. By 1968, the sampling interval could be safely shortened to 12 h, and to even as little as an overnight urine collection, which additionally gave greater comfort to a patient's life. A creatinine measure was still used to adjust for a complete day's output. Estrogen excretion remains fairly constant throughout the day, and the main gonadotropic effect would be expected within the first 8 h following an evening administration.

Prior to the widespread commercial availability of gonadotropins, only a small number of physicians benefitted from exclusive hormone distributions by the Serono Corporation. These individuals helped start the "Gonadotropin Club" (G-Club) which proposed the term HMG as well as the definitions of the First, and then the Second, International Reference Preparations (IRP) of HMG. Early members of the G Club included A. Netter and R. Palmer (Paris) and I. Bernard (Bordeaux) in France, and G.S. Jones in the USA [9].

Use of gonadotropins gradually increased through the 1960s albeit still at a limited rate. Statistical evaluation was not yet feasible because the few clinicians who were willing to attempt HMG stimulation were typically unable to present more than a few patients at scientific conferences. Discussions centered primarily on the safety range of estrogen levels, and optimal administration protocols (e.g., whether HMG should be administered daily or on alternate days, and how many vials should be used each time). The continuing major concern was how to provide adequate ovulation while minimizing the risk for hyperstimulation.

Other associated issues, that continue to be debated today, included:

- Whether a “slight” hyperstimulation might enhance the rate of successful pregnancy. It was argued that the range for the 12 h urine estrogen assay could safely be raised to 75–150 μg/24 h, which is significantly above physiologic preovulatory levels.
- The importance of the FSH/LH ratio in HMG. The ratio was typically close to 1 in the usual vials of *Pergonal*® or *Humegon*®, but Donini produced a *Neopergonal*® preparation in which FSH content could be been enriched from 2/1 to as much as 15/1 over LH content. Vials used in France during this time typically contained FSH/LH at 2/1, and provided satisfactory results [3]. However, although an FSH excess was not detrimental to ovarian stimulation, clinicians were reporting that preparations with an FSH/LH ratio of less than 1/1 had a tendency to provoke premature luteinization of the Graafian follicles.

Additional issues of concern included an occasionally severe hyperstimulation syndrome that could occur with estrogen levels well within the safety range, or that multiple pregnancies resulted in some instances where estrogen levels were not different from typical single pregnancies.

The availability of rapid plasma estradiol radioimmunoassay technology in the 1970s shed some light on these questions. Urine excretion of total estrogen is of course delayed in contrast to plasma levels and, although there is good overall correlation during periods of steady hormone secretion, a rapid rise in plasma might not be reflected in urine until the following day (Figs. 1.1 and 1.2). Thus a normal urine value (representing output during the previous night) could be observed while a spike of blood estrogen was occurring from a rapidly developing ovarian hyperstimulation. In response to this, Delafontaine and Grenier proposed a protocol modification designed to reduce risk for hyperstimulation and multiple pregnancy, namely to stop the HMG administration when the plasma estradiol level reached the safety range, and to administer hCG only when estrogen levels actually began to decrease (Fig. 1.3). This became the beginning of the concept of “coasting.” [4].

Reliable and sensitive assay techniques that used radioiodine tracers after extraction appeared in 1984–1985. A direct assay method using ^{131}I appeared in 2000, followed by the enzyme-linked immunoassays in 2002 that remain in use today. At the present time, measures of plasma estradiol by immunoassay is a simple, rapid procedure that reports a result within a very few hours of sampling, and daily secretion can be monitored, as desired.

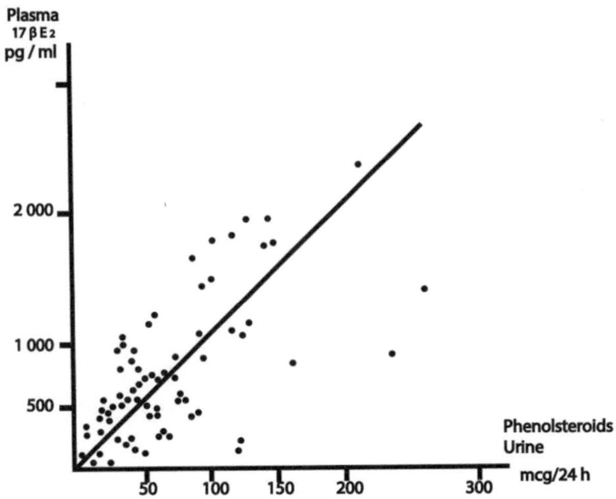

Fig. 1.1 Concordance of urinary and plasma estrogen levels (Courtesy of A. Ruffié)

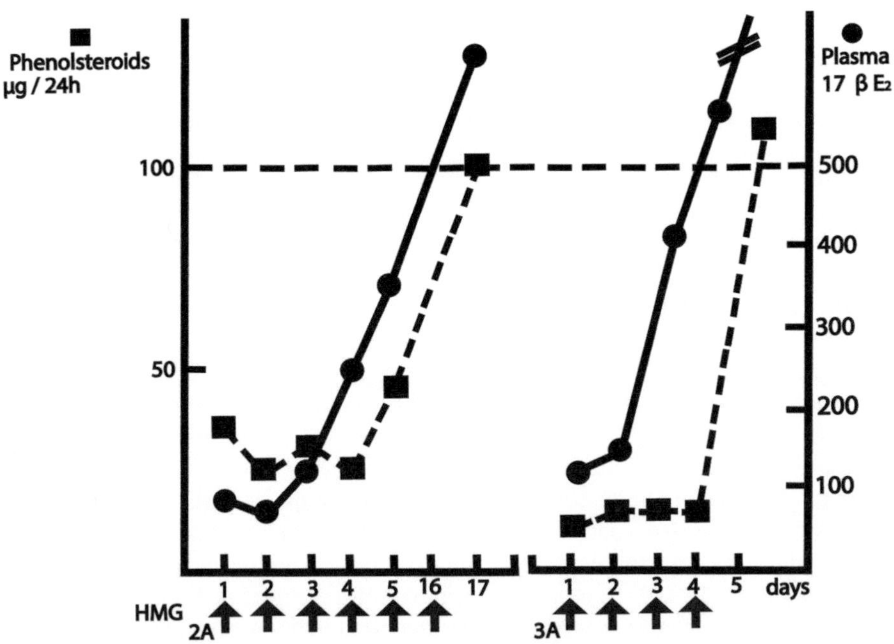

Fig. 1.2 Examples of two patients illustrating the potential for discrepancy between urinary and plasma estrogen assays that may occur when estradiol secretion is rising rapidly (Courtesy A. Ruffié)

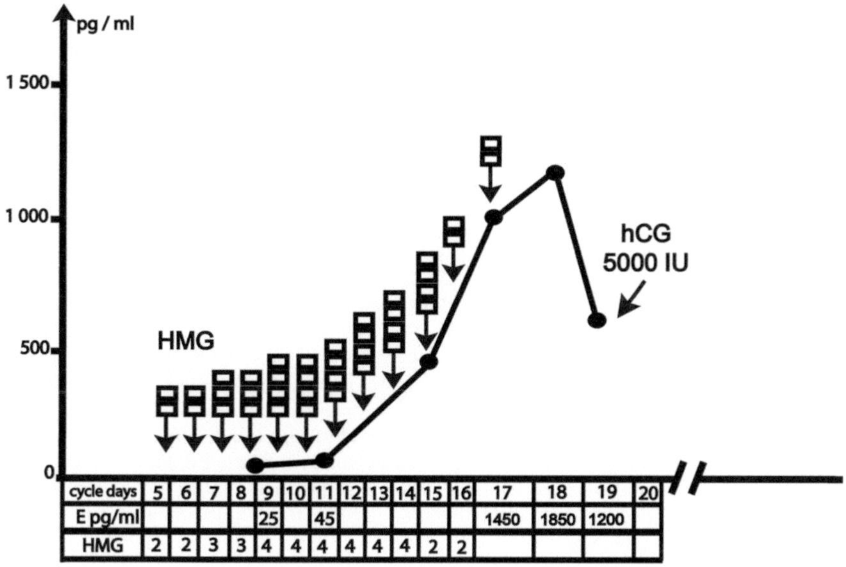

Fig. 1.3 A proposed protocol to reduce the risk of ovarian hyperstimulation and multiple pregnancy. Daily HMG injections are halted when plasma E_2 has risen sufficiently, and hCG is administered only after the E_2 level begins to decline [4]

1.2.2 Monitoring by Morphology

The final important advance for monitoring was the appearance of ultrasound imagery. Introduced into gynecology practice near the end of the 1970s, this procedure provides direct observation of the number, location, diameter and appearance of the developing ovarian follicle(s) [10]. With this technology it was soon revealed that similar plasma estradiol levels can occur with a variety of follicular situations, for instance, with one dominant follicle and a few smaller ones, or several mid-sized follicles, or with numerous small follicles.

In essence, ultrasound identifies best the risk for multiple pregnancy, while rapid estradiol measures guard best against risk for hyperstimulation [11]. Ultrasound imagery also permits estimation of endometrial grade and thickness, the amount of cervical mucus, and also of the ovarian reserve of antral follicles during in the early days of the cycle. It is still too soon to know whether an automated 3-dimensional count of all developing follicles will improve accuracy and safety even more, compared to the usual manual measurements.

There is no doubt that the combination of functional (plasma estradiol) and morphologic (ultrasound) criteria provides the optimal assurance of both efficacy and safety for an ovarian stimulation. In addition, measures of plasma LH and/or progesterone may help to identify the exact timing of ovulation for cases of intrauterine insemination, or when only a single intercourse is possible. LH data are also important when monitoring a controlled ovarian hyperstimulation (COH) for IVF purposes with a GnRH antagonist protocol. Some claims have been made that conducting only hormonal or only ultrasound monitoring, or even neither, can suffice for an adequate stimulation leading to IVF, but no feasibility study has successfully challenged the necessity of a using both hormonal and ultrasound for optimal monitoring of ovarian stimulation in the routine practice of reproductive medicine.

References

1. Brown JB (1978) Pituitary control of ovarian function. Concepts derived from gonadotropin therapy. Aust N Z J Obstet Gynaecol 18:47–54
2. Lunenfeld B, Rabau E, Rummey G, Winkelsberg G (1961) The responsiveness of the human ovary to gonadotropins (Hypophysis III). Proc Third World Congress Gynecol Obstet (Vienna) 1:220
3. Donini P (1968) Action de FSH et de LH sur la stimulation folliculaire. Définition du Neo-Pergonal. In: Les Gonadotrophines d'origine humaine. Byla-Searle Ed, Paris
4. Grenier J, Delafontaine D, Cornier E et al (1981) Régulation de l'induction de l'ovulation par l'association HMG-HCG. In: Hormonologie de la Stérilité – Explorations et Thérapeutique. SEPE Ed, Paris, pp 583–618
5. Ludwig M, Felberbaum RE, Diedrich K, Lunenfeld B (2002) Ovarian stimulation: from basic science to clinical application. Reprod Biomed Online 5(Suppl 1):73–86
6. Lunenfeld B, Sulimovici L, Rabau E, Eshkol A (1962) L'induction de l'ovulation dans les aménorrhées hypophysaires par un traitement combiné de gonadotrophines urinaires ménopausiques et de gonadotrophines chorioniques. C R Soc Fr Gyncol 32:346
7. Sagle MA, Hamilton Fairley D, Kiddy D, Franks S (1991) A comparative randomized study of low-dose human menopausal gonadotropin and follicle stimulating hormone in women with polycystic ovarian syndrome. Fertil Steril 55:56–60
8. Dubecq JP, Labadie P, Mathieu H, Ruffie A (1962) Modification apportée à la réaction colorée des phénolstéroïdes urinaire selon Ittrich. Bull Soc Pharm Bordeaux 101:159–188
9. Bernard I, Ruffie A (1973) Notre expérience des traitements modernes des stérilités par trouble de l'ovulation et les risques d'hyperstimulation. Bord Med 6:2549–2557
10. Hackloer DJ, Fleming R, Robinson HP et al (1979) Correlation of ultrasonic and endocrinologic assessment of human follicular development. Am J Obstet Gynecol 133:122–128
11. Emperaire JC, Vella M, Ruffie A (1982) Apport de l'échographie ovarienne dans la surveillance de l'induction de l'ovulation. Ses rapports avec la surveillance hormonale. Rev Franç Endocrinol Clin 23:379–384

2 Review of Physiology

The principal objective of mono- or paucifollicular ovarian stimulation is to improve or restore ovulation for a patient in which the process is occurring improperly or not at all, or to rescue additional follicles from atresia. On the other hand, a multifollicular stimulation is by its nature disruptive to normal ovarian function because it promotes maturation and development of abnormally numerous follicles. For this reason, it would appear useful to review briefly a few essential concepts of physiology as a way to orient thoughts on the logic, consistency and protocols of different approaches to ovulation stimulation.

At the heart of this process lies the relationship between the ovary and the anterior pituitary gland. The pituitary itself is controlled from the hypothalamus through its gonadotropin releasing hormone (GnRH, gonadorelin) that is in turn subject to influences from multiple areas of the central nervous system that express varied forms of external stimulation upon the pituitary-ovarian axis. Ovarian follicles secrete steroid hormones that act on their respective peripheral hormonal receptors, and they additionally exert feedback actions on the hypothalamic-pituitary complex.

2.1 The Anterior Pituitary-Ovarian Axis

Throughout her reproductive life, a woman's reserve of primordial follicles declines with advancing age, from some 200,000 at puberty to less than 1,000 at menopause. Each primordial follicle contains an oocyte resting in meiotic prophase I. The fate of a follicle destined for ovulation is actually decided 3 months earlier, when it is "awakened" from this primordial pool. Together with several others, it commences a slow maturation process under the influence of paracrine factors until arriving at the pre-antral stage, a crossing point controlled by anti-Müllerian hormone (AMH). At this point the targeted follicles acquire FSH receptors for the first time. Whereas previous growth was FSH-independent, the structures now become hormonally dependent. By the start of a menstrual cycle, several pre-antral follicles, each 2–5 mm in diameter, have survived the sequence of events during this "awakening" period (Fig. 2.1).

J.-C. Emperaire, *Ovulation Stimulation with Gonadotropins*,
DOI 10.1007/978-3-319-18654-2_2

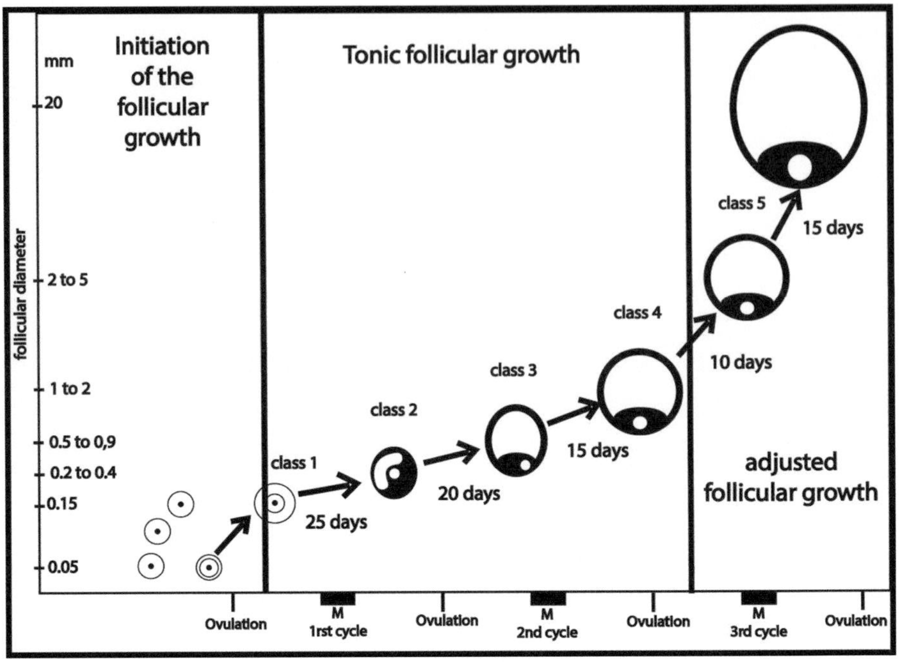

Fig. 2.1 Development of the ovarian follicle from the primordial stage through ovulation

As the menstrual cycle terminates, corpus luteal decay results in a fall of estrogen and progestin secretion that triggers a chain of endometrial changes leading to menstruation. This decline of steroids and inhibin A removes their inhibitory effects on the hypothalamic-pituitary axis and permits a rise of FSH that is perceptible in plasma even before the first day of the menstruation.

Enhanced secretion of FSH, at the end of the previous cycle and during the subsequent early follicular phase, stimulates pre-antral follicles inconsistently because the sensitivity of each follicle is correlated with its respective endowment of FSH receptors. As the growing wave of FSH surpasses the threshold of the most hormone-sensitive follicles, a period of rapid growth ensues for those recruited early, and an "FSH window" opens. With concomitant stimulation by pituitary LH, cells of the theca interna deliver an androgen substrate to the aromatase complex of adjacent granulosa cells that will synthetize increasing amounts of estradiol and also the protein hormone inhibin B. Estradiol in turn furthers the synthesis of additional FSH receptors, with assistance from FSH itself. This "snowballing" effect amplifies follicular sensitivity to both gonadotropins and enhances growth of follicles to the antral stage that is evidenced by accumulating follicular fluid. At the same time, estradiol and FSH induce the synthesis of LH receptors on the granulosa cells, thereby promoting still more estrogen secretion.

The few follicles recruited at the beginning of the cycle are asynchronous with the others as a result of their unique sensitivity to FSH. Although initially indistinguishable morphologically from other follicles, the one whose FSH threshold is lowest begins to grow before the others. Its aromatase complex is the first to be aroused by FSH, and it begins to secrete estrogens before the others. This follicle is then enabled to enter the "snowball" phase ahead of the remaining cohort and is becoming the "selected one" to yield a gamete. As the other follicles join to secrete increasing amounts of estradiol and inhibin B, a negative feedback begins to impact pulsatile FSH release at the hypothalamic-pituitary level. On about the seventh day of the menstrual cycle, FSH secretion falls and the "FSH window" closes. Only the selected follicle continues growing, thanks to its rich population of FSH receptors that permits development even in the face of declining FSH. Whereas growth of all the remaining less sensitive follicles diminishes or stops altogether during the late follicular phase, the lead follicle, now 1 cm in diameter, expands due to additional stimulation from an FSH-like effect of LH. The aromatase complex also becomes functionally coupled to LH receptors, permitting additional LH participation in the selected follicle's primacy and its late follicular phase maturation. By this time all of the other irregularly stimulated follicles that were initially recruited at the beginning of the cycle have undergone atresia and vanish within the ovarian stroma.

When plasma estradiol levels have been maintained in excess of 100 pg/ml for more than 48 h, and when the selected follicular diameter begins to exceed 16 mm, a large release of hypothalamic GnRH elicits a surge of pituitary FSH and LH. This final gonadotropin wave initiates a stream of follicular events leading to an initial erosion of the follicular wall accompanied by an increase of follicular fluid osmotic pressure that provokes a triad of events: a follicular rupture at the apex, a differentiation of the cumulus, and a final maturation of the oocyte itself. The oocyte's meiotic process is awakened from prophase I through metaphase II, where maturation is again halted to await arrival of a haploid spermatozoon.

Following expulsion of the ovum, the follicle's remaining granulosa cells become heavily vascularized and join with remaining theca interna to be transformed into luteinized cells. The corpus luteum actively secretes estradiol accompanied by a large output of progesterone, all being directed by a pulsatile signal from pituitary LH. Luteal lifespan is already programmed for 12–14 days unless its function can be rescued and maintained by exponentially rising chorionic gonadotropin (hCG) levels from trophoblast of an implanting embryo. While the menstrual cycle progressively develops under the influence of two pituitary gonadotropins, FSH and LH, the third gonadotropin, hCG, of placental origin, appears once the embryo implants. This signals the transformation of a menstrual cycle into a beginning pregnancy.

2.2 Follicle-Stimulating Hormone (FSH)

Throughout the menstrual cycle, follicle-stimulating hormone is secreted in a pulsatile manner by gonadotrophs in the adenohypophysis, a process that is itself controlled through a pulsatile release of hypothalamic gonadorelin (GnRH). FSH is delivered through blood to specific receptors on the surface of the ovarian granulosa cells and act to promote follicular growth and development. Despite a modest degradation by the liver, and elimination from the body by the kidneys, urinary FSH retains its biological activity (i.e., it is still able to bind to, and activate, ovarian receptors).

The evolution of ovarian follicles is directed by substantial changes of plasma FSH levels throughout the menstrual cycle. Levels are highest during the end of the luteal phase and early follicular phase (the recruitment period). Then FSH begins to decrease in mid-follicular phase (the selection-leadership period) due to the negative feedback effect of rising levels of estradiol and inhibin B (Fig. 2.2). There is a pre-ovulatory surge of FSH, synchronous with the LH surge, and then levels enter a declining period, only to rise again at the end of the luteal phase.

The physiologic role of FSH is directed solely toward proliferation and development of ovarian granulosa cells, thereby to control follicular growth. FSH also induces secretion of inhibin B and, together with estradiol, the appearance and proliferation of LH receptors in the follicle. Finally the pre-ovulatory FSH peak participates importantly in the maturation of the cumulus-oocyte complex.

2.2.1 FSH: A Complex Molecule

Follicle-stimulating hormone is a heterodimer composed of alpha and beta subunits linked noncovalently. The alpha subunit is a chain of 92 amino acids folded by five disulfide bonds, and is identical to the alpha subunits of other glycoprotein hormones: thyrotropin (TSH), luteotropin (LH), and chorionic gonadotropin (hCG).

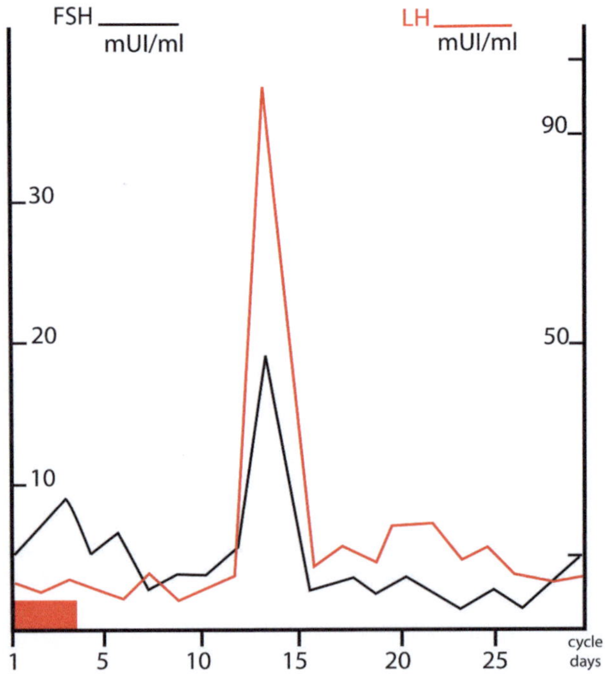

Fig. 2.2 Patterns of plasma FSH and LH throughout the menstrual cycle

The beta subunit of FSH is composed of 111 amino acids folded by six disulfide bonds. However, this structure, as with each of the glycoprotein hormones, is unique to its respective hormone. Neither subunit of FSH has biological activity; only the conjoined heterodimer is capable of expressing a hormonal response.

FSH molecules are also characterized by glycosylation: each subunit bears two oligosaccharide chains (glycans) linked to asparagine residues (Asn 52 and Asn 78 on the alpha subunit, Asn7 and Asn 24 on the beta-subunit). These saccharide chains are constructed of N-acetyl-glucosamine, monosaccharides (mannose, galactose), and terminal sialic acids that become more numerous through side-chain branching. Varied oligosaccharide branching results in a number of unique FSH isoforms, also known as isohormones or glycoforms [1]. The pattern of branching is responsible for their richness of sugars (glycosylation) and sialic acid (sialylation) (Fig. 2.3). The glycosylated chains are essential for the full expression of hormonal activity, and cleavage leads to a progressive decline of activity in target cells. The alpha subunit saccharide chains appear to be most important for FSH receptor activation and initiation of the intracellular signal transduction process (adenylate cyclase), whereas the beta subunit chains are known to play a major role in protecting the FSH molecule against degradation and elimination.

Some 20–30 FSH isoforms have been identified with distinctive oligosaccharide chain complexes that determine their ability to be maintained in circulation, to bind

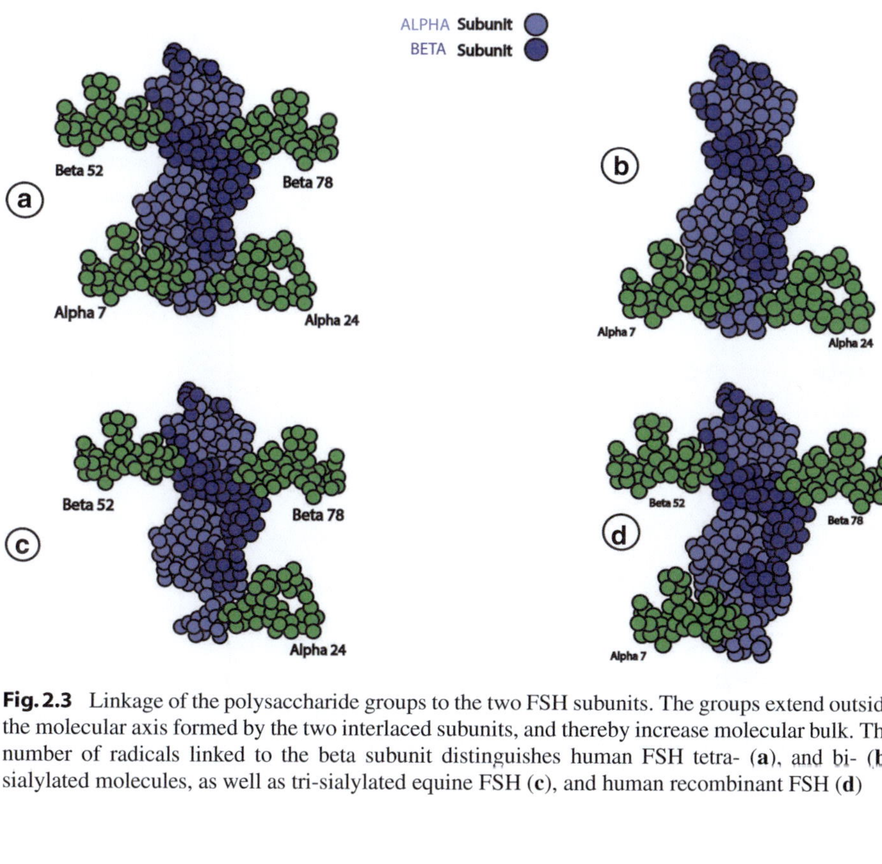

Fig. 2.3 Linkage of the polysaccharide groups to the two FSH subunits. The groups extend outside the molecular axis formed by the two interlaced subunits, and thereby increase molecular bulk. The number of radicals linked to the beta subunit distinguishes human FSH tetra- (**a**), and bi- (**b**) sialylated molecules, as well as tri-sialylated equine FSH (**c**), and human recombinant FSH (**d**)

to the FSH receptor, and to induce a biological response [2]. Observations that the mix of isoforms found in pituitary tissue and in plasma are identical suggest that circulating hormone is not simply the degradation product of a single secreted molecule [3]. Physicochemical characteristics of each isoform are determined by three parameters which affect their physiological properties (Fig. 2.4):

- Their degree of sialylation in relation to the number of the terminal sialic acid residues, in part a function of the oligosaccharide chain complexity.
- Their degree of sulfonation (sulfonic acid radicals): there is significant competition between galactosamine transferase and galactotransferase at the terminal N-acetylglucosamine residue of the common mucopolysaccharide core. The former attaches an N-acetylgalactosamine residue, followed by a terminal sulfonate, whereas the latter enzyme attaches a galactose residue followed by a terminal sialic acid. In contrast to pituitary LH, no FSH isoform contains more than two sulfonate radicals.
- Their degree of glycosaccharidic chain intricacy, in relation to the richness in chain branching and complexity, and particularly the presence of a bisecting N-acetylglucosamine radical between two other common core segments.

As the branch complexity of FSH isoforms increases, the molecules become more acidic, due to the lateral chains acquiring two to four terminal sialate radicals (or "antennas"). Isoforms are distinguishable by their sialic acid content which proportionately lowers the isoelectric point (pI). Natural FSH becomes a mixture of

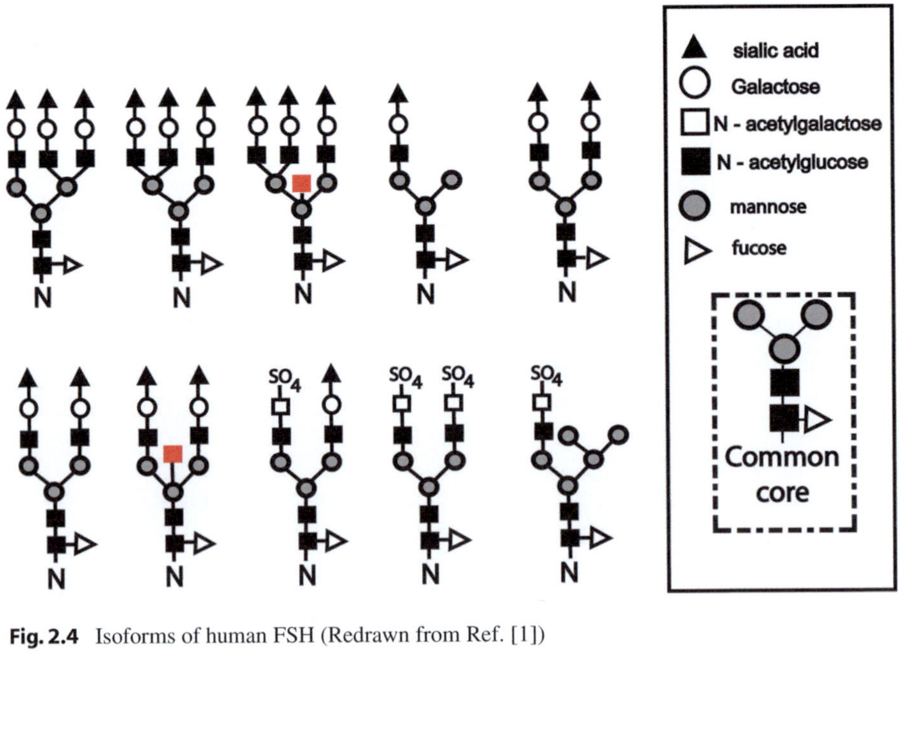

Fig. 2.4 Isoforms of human FSH (Redrawn from Ref. [1])

isoforms with isoelectric points between three (most acidic) and six (least acidic). Nevertheless, mere recognition and identification of the varied FSH isoforms based solely on pI is not in itself sufficient; the richness of internal branching and the number of "antennas" also plays an important part in bioactivity. Isoforms with varied oligosaccharide complexity or degree of sulfonation can share the same level of overall sialylation yet express distinct physiological properties.

Glycosylation of the FSH beta subunit is a separate issue. A portion of the subunit molecules have no glycosylation at either Asn 7 or Asn 24 which results in a mixture of tetra- (MW 24,000) and bi- (MW 21,000) sialylated molecules. This mixture is the result of the hormonal milieu in blood: estradiol decreases the rate of N-glycosylation, most likely through inhibition of oligosaccharyl transferase. Bi-glycosylated forms comprise 75–95 % of the molecular population in postmenopausal women, but only 35–40 % of plasma FSH in menstruating women [4]. This shift of proportion exerts important effects upon the 3-dimensional configuration of the FSH molecules, and hence upon plasma clearance. Both of the N-glycans of the alpha subunit are aligned along the molecule's axis, whereas the N-glycans of the beta subunit extend outward, effectively doubling the molecular diameter and reducing its rate of glomerular filtration. Studies of a mutant di-glycosylated recombinant FSH showed an elimination rate from blood to be twice as fast as that of normal tetra-glycosylated rFSH [5]. This "all or nothing" process of beta subunit glycosylation provides yet another control mechanism over bioactivity, plus it alters the electrical charge of the molecule as the proportion of the 2- and 4-glycan isoforms shifts. A final point: 3-glycosylated isoforms, having a single radical on the beta subunit (Asn 24), may be found in natural equine FSH or in recombinant human FSH (on Asn 7) but this is never found in naturally occurring human FSH.

The degree of sialylation, and of possible sulfonation, exerts a considerable influence on metabolism of the various isoforms. FSH metabolism begins with removal of hormone from plasma by binding to receptors for specific sialic acid or sulfated residues in hepatic epithelial cells, and followed by renal excretion. More numerous sialic residues on a molecule hinder its hepatic capture and slow its glomerular filtration due to the expanded molecular size. Consequently, the more sialylated and acidic isoforms persist in blood for a longer period. An isohormone with a pI of 4.27 has a half-life of 24 h, but the duration falls to 12 h for isoforms at a pI of 5.49 [6]. On the other hand, for the same degree of sialylation, the addition of sulfone radicals enhances the rate of extraction and elimination of the glycoforms, in direct proportion with the number of SO radicals [7]. Thus the pituitary actually secretes a mixture of isoforms, and each interacts uniquely with the ovarian FSH receptor.

In addition, the structural mix of secreted molecules is not static, and it changes throughout one's life. The mix also changes throughout the menstrual cycle in reproductive-age women, in accordance with GnRH pulsatility that is principally controlled by the plasma levels of estradiol. The more acidic FSH isoforms prevail during lower estrogen environments, such as before puberty and after menopause. Similarly, more acidic isoforms dominate at the beginning and the end of the menstrual cycle, and less acidic isohormones prevail during the pre-ovulatory period to produce a more homogenous distribution (Fig. 2.5) [8]. Individual patients secrete a uniquely tailored isoform profile that is already distinguishable on cycle day 3. The same occurs for LH isoforms [9].

Bioactivity of the isoforms also varies according to the model studied. Whereas in vivo activity is principally related to the molecular half-life, in vitro activity becomes more a function of its affinity for the cellular receptors. The relative activity of FSH isoforms is affected by their degree of glycosylation, in an apparently conflicting manner [10]:

- The more acidic glycoforms show a higher bioactivity in vivo, for example, in the Steelman-Pohley bioassay that measures a dose–response variation of immature rat ovarian weight in relation to the injected FSH doses.
- On the contrary, the less acidic isoforms show a higher affinity in vitro for the receptor, and thus a higher bioactivity that stimulates an earlier, more rapid and intense estradiol secretion by the granulosa cells, that may also be enhanced by a stronger postreceptor activity.

This outward inconsistency is explained, at least in part, by the clearance of the different isohormones, related itself to their degree of glycosylation. The more acidic forms are picked up and removed from the plasma more slowly, because of the sialic acid inhibition of FSH binding to the hepatic asialo-glycoproteic receptors: their prolonged existence within the blood stream partly compensates for their lower bioactivity.

It should be noted that both in vivo and in vitro assays measuring the FSH activity have their own limits. In vivo models fail to account for interspecies variations of FSH clearance, and for the possible bias introduced by a bolus injection of hormone that contrasts to the normal pulsatile secretion of FSH. On the other hand, in vitro assays, while avoiding the hormone half-life issues, measure only a single type of response, e.g., androgen aromatization by rat granulosa or Sertoli cells, or

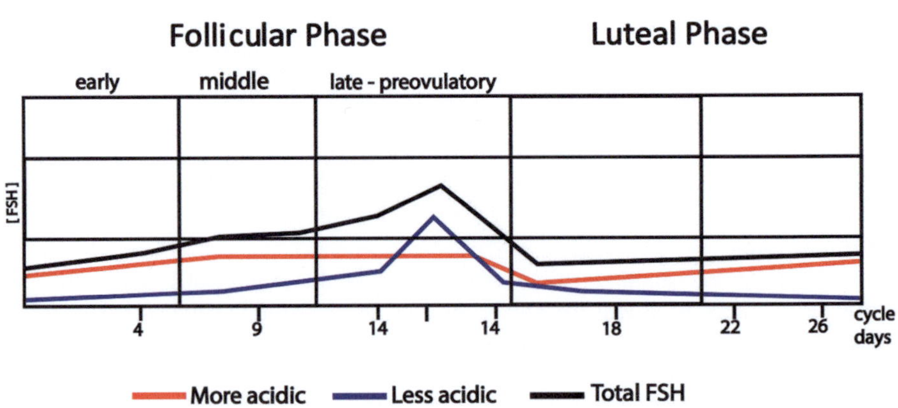

Fig. 2.5 Profile of FSH isoform secretion during the menstrual cycle (Redrawn from Ref. [2])

the quantity of AMP produced by cell lines expressing the human FSH receptor. Reliance on a single response parameter is unable to account for the intricacy of the complete follicular response to FSH, that includes follicular development, sequential as well as synergetic differentiation of granulosa and theca cells, antrum formation and antral fluid secretion. These concerns have raised awareness of working toward in vitro testing models that utilize intact ovarian follicles of mice capable of being grown to full maturity. This would lead to an improved evaluation of follicle and oocyte quality with respect to the various hormonal isoforms being tested.

It should be further noted that bioactivity differences between the different isoforms of FSH are not solely explained by their isoelectric point, but are also subject to individual properties that were revealed by in vitro studies of intact mouse follicles. Results from this model lend strength to the critical importance of FSH in antral follicular development, and also illustrate how all follicular cells – granulosa, theca and oocyte – are responding to increasing FSH dosages [11]:

- A rather precise threshold dose stimulates follicular antrum formation, which supports the concept of an FSH threshold often observed in clinical practice; no FSH effects are detectible below the threshold dose.
- A maximal dose above which degenerative modifications appear histologically in granulosa and theca cells, as well as in the oocyte. There appears to be a "ceiling" dose, over which granulosa cell death and oocyte damage has been observed, which characterizes a true FSH overdose, at least at the follicle level.
- An FSH "efficacy range" that occurs between the threshold and ceiling doses.

Importantly, these three parameters are known to vary widely according to the molecular isoform pI being tested. Less acidic glycohormones can provoke follicular growth at concentrations as low as 1.5 μg/ml, and can stimulate a follicular pool, even those less sensitive, yet their "ceiling" can be as low as 5 μg/ml. The more acidic isoforms, in contrast, are effective only at concentrations above 40 μg/ml, to an activity ceiling of 400 μg/ml. The latter isoform induces a more selective follicular growth. Similarly, a less acidic mixture of FSH isohormones stimulates a more rapid follicular growth in vitro. Additionally, use of this model makes it possible to follow different isoform effects up through the overall embryo quality, beginning with the oocyte of a chosen follicle.

All these varied data confirm a higher bioactivity of the less acidic isoform, and explain further the relevance of the spectrum of composition changes in the FSH secreted throughout the menstrual cycle. Follicular recruitment occurs under the effect of relatively high quantities of more acidic isoforms that have a higher activity threshold and larger efficacy range. Dominance of less acidic isoforms in the middle and late follicular phases serves to increase estrogen secretion and stimulate granulosa cell mitosis, which enhances the overall FSH effect on antral development.

This mouse model also underscores the concept that the different source-related bioactivities of FSH cannot be attributed solely to variations of isoelectric point.

When the in vitro responses of an intact follicle to natural pituitary FSH are compared to those of recombinant FSH normalized to the same pI (3.5–5.3), the threshold dose is lower for rFSH. This higher in vitro bioactivity cannot be explained by charge discrepancies between the isoforms of the two preparations. Perhaps the use of a nonhuman cell line for rFSH synthesis results in other subtle consequences for bioactivity that would be located within the specific glycosaccharidic chain structure and composition.

There is also growing evidence that, in addition to pI differences, various FSH isoforms might play a specific role in the recruitment, and then development, of the dominant follicle up to the moment of ovulation, as is known to be the case for LH, and that this has some noticeable outcomes on the embryo quality. In vitro, some glycoforms show a particular ability to stimulate estradiol secretion, or granulosa cell proliferation, or even synthesis of plasminogen that is crucial in the optimal maturation of the pre-ovulatory follicle and its wall dehiscence. Other isohormones are endowed with paradoxical properties, such as an LH-like effect or a FSH antagonist activity. At some future time therapeutic FSH molecules may be tailored by procedures that shorten one or several carefully selected isoforms [12].

2.2.2 The FSH Receptor

FSH exerts its activity through specific receptors located on the surface of ovarian granulosa cells. These guanine nucleotide-binding, signal-transducing proteins (often called G protein-coupled receptors or GPR) are constructed of extracellular, transmembrane, and intracellular domains (Fig. 2.6). A receptor's primary sequence is susceptible to genomic variations. Aside from uncommon mutations that result in loss of sensitivity to FSH, more numerous variants can have significant implications for clinical practice. Many receptor polymorphisms are as simple as an alteration of a single DNA nucleotide (single nucleotide polymorphism, or SNP), and can occur in at least 1 % of all people. Among the more clinically significant polymorphisms, allelic combinations at position 680 are of clinical importance; the heterozygous asparagin/serin (Asn/Ser) mutation, however, is more widespread than the homozygous variants Ser/Ser and Asn/Asn [13]:

- The Ser/Ser genotype produces a receptor having decreased sensitivity to FSH that leads to a slightly elevated plasma level, and the necessity for higher FSH doses to drive ovarian stimulation [14];
- The Asn/Asn genotype, on the contrary, can induce an exaggerated sensitivity to FSH that could enhance the risk for severe ovarian hyperstimulation [15].

Taken together, normally-occurring polymorphisms of both the FSH molecular isoforms and of the FSH receptor are likely responsible for many of the varied responses of the same patient to the different available FSH preparations, as well as the different outcomes between patients receiving the same FSH preparation.

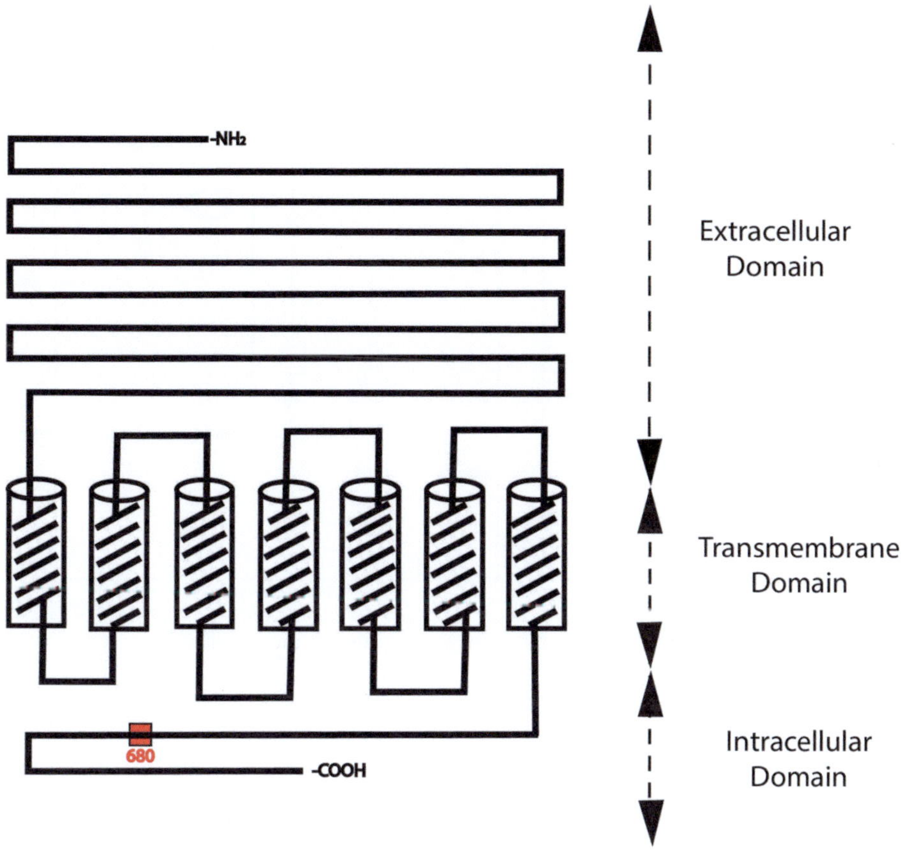

Fig. 2.6 Structure of the FSH receptor (Redrawn from Ref. [1])

2.2.3 Mechanisms of Action

Overall, pituitary FSH is the main hormone responsible for ovarian follicular development. There are four aspects to its action:

1. *The two-compartment theory*: The long-held belief that the follicle comprises distinct anatomical and functional compartments (Fig. 2.7) has never been seriously challenged.

- Granulosa cells are simulated by FSH to synthesize the aromatase complex, and also inhibin B, a hormone that in turn diminishes FSH secretion at the hypothalamic-pituitary level.
- Theca Interna cells are stimulated by LH to produce androgens that migrate toward the avascular granulosa component and are converted to estrogens by FSH-stimulated aromatase. Estradiol then acts locally, along with ovarian para-

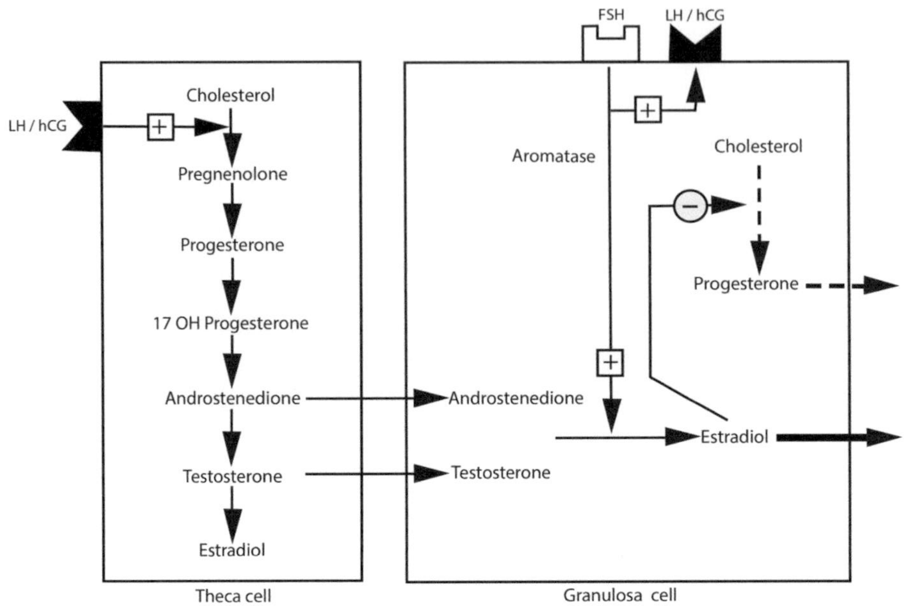

Fig. 2.7 Steroidogenesis during the follicular phase in the distinct compartments of theca and granulosa cells

crine factors, to increase the population of estrogen receptors in granulosa cells, and thus to enhance follicular sensitivity to this hormone. Estradiol discharged into the bloodstream signals numerous peripheral as well as CNS sites, in particular uterine and cervical mucosa, as the dominant follicle reaches maturity.

2. *The FSH threshold*: Each small antral follicle has a unique sensitivity to FSH, generally related to its original receptor population. Accordingly, this sensitivity varies among different follicles (Fig. 2.8).

- For each follicle, the FSH threshold is adjusted by plasma hormone levels that start its development.
- For a pool of follicles, the FSH threshold is the plasma level required to commence growth of the most sensitive follicles. When FSH levels rise above this threshold even if only 10–30 %, the growth of lesser sensitive follicles becomes progressively stimulated.

3. *The FSH window*: This is the period of time when plasma FSH remains above its threshold level, initiating and supporting development of growing follicles. The window then closes when FSH levels recede beneath the threshold. At this point new growth is arrested, and atresia begins in those partially developed follicles that were less sensitive to FSH (Fig. 2.8).

These final two parameters may be manipulated with intention. For example, if one seeks multiple follicular development and ovulation for in vitro fertilization, initial administration of higher FSH doses that rapidly increase plasma levels above the threshold will result in an enhanced follicular recruitment.

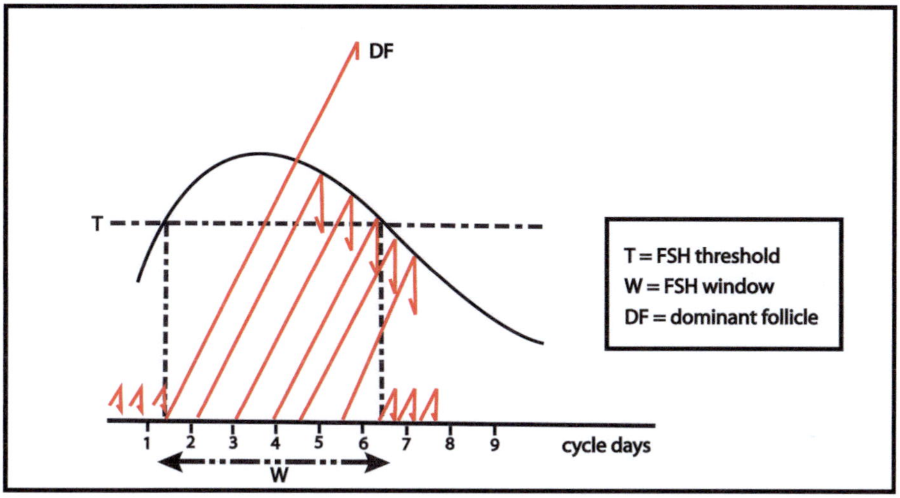

Fig. 2.8 Illustration of the FSH threshold (*T*) and window (*W*)

Maintenance of elevated FSH levels throughout the stimulation process prevents the window from closing and leads to development and maturity of a significant number of recruited follicles. On the other hand, if one seeks a more classical stimulation to grow and mature a single follicle, it becomes crucial to respect the basic principles that govern the more physiological monofollicular cycle.

4. *FSH molecular structure*: Despite the fact that secreted FSH has been long recognized to be a collection of distinct isoform molecules, whose composition varies throughout the menstrual cycle, enhanced interest in these different isohormones has appeared only recently. Hopefully this interest will result in a continued sophistication of ovarian stimulation protocols.

2.3 Luteinizing Hormone (LH)

Like FSH, LH is a heterodimer. It is composed of a 92-amino acid alpha subunit that is identical to FSH-α, and a covalently bound unique 121 amino acid beta subunit (Fig. 2.9). LH is much less sialylated than FSH or chorionic gonadotropin (hCG) and has a less acidic isoelectric point in the range of 7.1–9.5. Both di- and tri- glycosylated isoforms are present in serum [16]. Some 17 LH glycoforms have been identified by pI from pituitary tissue. As is the case for FSH, the clearance rate from blood of the different LH isoforms is hindered in proportion to their degree of sialylation, and accelerated by the degree of sulfonation. Also similarly to FSH, LH binding affinity to its receptor, and resulting in vitro bioactivity, decreases, and plasma half-life increases, as the pI declines. The least

Alpha subunit (92aa) ALA ———— ASN (52) ———— ASN (78) ———— SER — COOH

Beta subunit LH (121 aa) SER ———— ASN (30) ———— LEU – COOH

Beta subunit hCG (145 aa) SER — ASN (13) — ASN (30) — SER (121) — SER (127) — SER (132) — SER (138) — GLN – COOH

Beta subunit FSH (118 aa) ASP —— ASN (7) —— ASN (24) ———— GLU – COOH

Fig. 2.9 Essential features of primary structures of the common alpha subunit and unique beta subunits of FSH, LH, and hCG

acidic isoforms are some 16 times more bioactive than the most acidic isoforms, due to enhanced receptor binding, and despite a slower clearance of the latter.

Less acidic LH isoforms have fewer oligosaccharide moieties, typically containing only one "antenna" with a terminal mannose residue; the more acidic glycoforms have more complex oligosaccharide chains, often with two "antennae" having sialic acid or N-galactosamine sulfate terminals. Desialylation of the LH molecule reduces in vivo bioactivity by over 100-fold, but without affecting immunoactivity [17].

The mix of plasma LH isoforms also changes throughout the menstrual cycle, being less acidic during the pre-ovulatory surge peak (pI of 8.0–9.0) than during either the follicular or luteal phases (7.5–8.9) [2]. Di-glycosylated LH circulates at lower concentrations than the triglycosylated form throughout the menstrual cycle, except at midcycle when the opposite occurs [16]. Isoform profiles are also very distinctive for each person [18].

The mix of LH isohormones in urine contrasts with plasma, due to the variable rates of renal clearance as well as to the effects of chemical purification procedures used in hormone extraction. When two pharmaceutical preparations of HMG were on the market, the Humegon® isoform mix was much less acidic than the Pergonal® mix.

LH acts through a specific receptor, also activated by hCG (LH/hCG receptor, LHr), located on cells of the ovarian theca interna, granulosa and in the corpus luteum. This receptor belongs to the same G-coupled superfamily as the FSH receptor, and has the typical composition of extra-cellular, intra-cellular, and transmembrane domains. It shares approximately a 50 % homology with the FSH receptor. Primordial and primary follicles are devoid of LHr, which begin to appear on granulosa and theca cells when antral follicles reach a 0.3 mm size. Receptor population then increases as the follicles mature to the pre-ovulatory stage, and LHr protein appears also to be expressed in the cumulus cells. LHr protein is ubiquitously present in the corpus luteum. Receptor development does not seem to occur simultaneously, but gradually at different times and in varied follicular sizes. Only a subset of follicles produce LHr at sufficient levels to enable response to administered hCG, which may explain why all of the oocytes are not equally mature at the time of aspiration for IVF [19].

The physiologic role of LH in ovarian function varies according to the target:

- In the theca interna of growing follicles, LH stimulates the synthesis of androgens. While some product is secreted into the bloodstream, most of the androgen production moves toward the granulosa cells to become a substrate for estrogen biosynthesis by the aromatase complex.
- In granulosa cells of the growing follicle, expression of the LH/hCG receptor is apparently controlled by FSH action. In essence LH and FSH synergistically promote final maturation of the dominant follicle.
- In mature follicles, the pre-ovulatory surge of LH initiates a chain of irreversible events within the follicle and its contents, leading to its rupture and expulsion of its gamete. Pre-ovulatory transformations of the cumulus cells are provoked together with the concomitant FSH surge.
- In the corpus luteum, a pulsatile secretion of pituitary LH supports the postovulatory release of estradiol and progesterone for 12–14 days.

In addition, alterations of the LH molecule or of its secretion patterns may serve to explain certain clinical abnormalities

- LH levels are frequently elevated in the polycystic ovary syndrome, due to a basal hypersecretion through an increased pulse frequency and amplitude, that is only partly compensated by a preferential secretion of less acidic LH isoforms having a shorter half-life [20].
- One of the genetic variants of LH has two mutations in the beta subunit, one of which contains an additional glycosylated radical that increases its half-life. This tends to diminish LH pulsatility, which could explain the excessive rate of ovulatory disorders and idiopathic infertility that occurs more commonly in these patients [21].
- A common polymorphic allele of the LH beta-subunit (V-beta LH) is associated with higher FSH consumption during controlled ovarian stimulation for assisted reproductive technology [22].

Overall, LH has an essential role in the ovarian steroidogenesis, as well as a secondary role in the final maturation of the follicle. Unfortunately, the fact that hCG has the same biological profile as LH in the most essential clinical indications has retarded important advances in understanding the properties and possible clinical advantages of the different LH isoforms.

2.4 Human Chorionic Gonadotropin (hCG)

hCG is secreted by the placenta throughout the entire pregnancy, from implantation to delivery. There are also reports of minute, pulsatile secretions of pituitary hCG together with pulses of LH. However, these are detectible only with high plasma LH concentration, such as during the pre-ovulatory gonadotropin surge and after menopause. Indeed, the gene coding for the LH beta subunit is located among the seven genes coding for hCG beta. In contrast to FSH and LH, hCG is not produced as a single molecule, but as several molecules; some variants have no hormonal activity. The total product secreted by placental trophoblast and by nontrophoblastic tumors, includes five distinct hCG molecules [23]:

Complete hCG, a heterodimer of two covalently-bound subunits.

The alpha subunit (identical to FSH and LH α) is a single 92-amino acid chain with two glycosaccharidic chains bound to Asn residues, and with two or three "antennae."

The beta subunit, specific to hCG and composed of 155 amino acids, has two Asn-bound glycosaccharidic chains having two or three "antennae" each. The primary sequence of the first 121 N-terminal amino acids is very close to that of the LH-ß subunit, but hCG-β has an additional 34 amino acids at the C-terminal end (carboxyl terminal peptide, CTP). This additional sequence also contains four tri- or hexa-saccharide chains O-linked to serine residues. The presence of these residues results in a higher volume of distribution for hCG, and a prolonged presence in blood.

Hyperglycosylated hCG: This is the complete hCG molecule bearing additional trisaccharide N-linked chains and hexasaccharide O-linked chains. Its molecular weight reaches 40,000 (versus 36,000 for the complete hCG), of which 25–30 % of the total MW is oligosaccharide.

Three unpaired subunits: Also secreted are free alpha and beta hyperglycosylated subunits and a free O-glycosylated alpha subunit. These unpaired alpha subunits are devoid of biological activity.

Placental syncytiotrophoblast secretes the whole hCG and the free alpha subunits, whereas the hyperglycosylated hCG and the free O-glycosylated alpha subunits are produced by the cytotrophoblast cells.

The degradation of the whole hCG begins in plasma under the effect of circulating macrophage proteases. Alpha and beta subunits are first separated, and then each is further cleaved. One large cleavage unit is the unique CTP chain at amino acids 93–155 on the beta subunit. Freed subunits and hydrolysis products are cleared from the plasma ten times faster than the whole dimeric hCG, particularly when the CTP group has been cleaved. Plasma of pregnant woman may contain up to ten degradation products in addition to the five complete hCG molecules originally synthesized. None of the degradation products is biologically active.

As a result, extracted urinary hCG is a highly heterogeneous mix of 15 distinct molecules resulting from renal degradation. A commonly found structure is a core fragment of the beta subunit containing two sequences (amino acids 6–40 and 55–92) still bound together by five disulfide bridges. The proportion of this beta-core fragment rises throughout pregnancy and by the seventh week of gestation can actually exceed levels of the whole bioactive hCG in urine. This biologically inactive material is typically the dominant hCG-related molecule in urine by the time of parturition.

The physiologic action of hCG is notable by having a higher, more stable affinity for the LH/hCG receptor than does LH, because of its enhanced glycosylation. In addition, the prolonged half-life (24–33 h for the slow elimination period, versus 10–12 h for LH) explains the more robust in vivo biological effect that is, for example, seven times higher in the rat seminal vesicle assay (a target for Leydig cell androgen production); it also explains the unique physiologic roles of each hormone [24].

It has always been believed that the physiological role of hCG is relegated to stimulation of progesterone production by ovarian luteal cells during early pregnancy, but it has never seemed logical that a hormone produced for 37 weeks should exist for only a 3-week span until the placenta's own progesterone production becomes adequate. Indeed, numerous additional basic actions of hCG have been highlighted during the past decade, including support for angiogenesis of the myometrial spiral cells, and fusion of the syncytio- and cytotrophoblast cells. Both actions are critical functions for a normal placentation that could have become involved in the brain development throughout human evolution [23].

References

1. Ulloa-Aguirre A, Timossi C (1998) Structure-function relationship of follicle-stimulating hormone and its receptor. Hum Reprod Update 4:260–283
2. Stanton PG, Burgon PG, Hearn MTW, Mendez JP (1996) Structural and functional characterization of FSH and LH isoforms. Mol Cell Endocrinol 125:133–141
3. Ulloa-Aguirre A, Timossi C, Mendez JP (2001) Is there any physiological role for gonadotropin oligosaccharide hetrogenicity in human? I. Gonadotropins are synthesized and released in multiple molecular forms. A matter of fact. Hum Reprod 16:599–604
4. Bousfield GR, Butnev VY, Walton W et al (2007) All-or-none N-glycosylation in primate follicle stimulating hormone ß-subunits. Mol Cell Endocrinol 262:40–48
5. D'Antonio M, Borrelli F, Datola A et al (1999) Biological characterization of recombinant human follicle stimulating hormone isoforms. Hum Reprod 14:1160–1167
6. Timossi CM, Barrios-di-Tomassi J, Gonzalez-Suarez R et al (2000) Differentiated effects of the charge variants of human follicle stimulating hormone. J Endocrinol 165:193–205
7. Wide L, Eriksson K, Sluss PM, Hall JE (2009) Serum half-life of pituitary gonadotropins is decreased by sulfonation and increased by sialylation in women. J Clin Endocrinol Metab 94:958–964
8. Anobile CJ, Talbot JA, McCann SJ et al (1998) Glycoform composition of serum gonadotropins through the normal menstrual cycle and in the post-menopause state. Mol Hum Reprod 4:631–639
9. Phillips DJ, Albertson-Xikland K, Eriksson K et al (1997) Changes in the isoform of luteinizing hormone and follicle stimulating hormone during puberty in normal children. J Clin Endocrinol Metab 82:3103–3106
10. Ryan RJ, Charlesworth MC, McCormick DJ, Milius RP et al (1982) The glycoprotein hormones: recent studies of structure-function relationship. FASEB J 2:2661–2669
11. Nayudu P, Vitt UA, Barrios de Tomasi J et al (2002) Intact follicle culture: what it can tell us about the roles of glycoforms during the follicle development. Reprod Biomed Online 5:240–253
12. Emperaire JC (2011) Propriétés et intérêt clinique des isoformes de la FSH. MT Med Reprod Gynecol Endocrinol 13:49–60
13. Hughes JN (2011) Récepteur de la FSH et stimulation ovarienne. In: Franchin R (ed) La stimulation ovarienne: concepts et réalités. MED'COM, Paris, p 41

14. Perez Mayorga M, Gromoll J, Behre HM et al (2000) Ovarian response to follicle stimulating hormone (FSH) stimulation depends on the FSH receptor genotype. J Clin Endocrinol 85:3365–3369
15. Daelmans C, Smits G, de Maertelaer V et al (2004) Prediction of severity of symptoms in iatrogenic ovarian hyperstimulation syndrome by follicle stimulating hormone receptor Ser680Asn polymorphism. J Clin Endocrinol Metab 89:6310–6315
16. Wide L, Eriksson K (2013) Dynamic changes in glycosylation and glycan composition of human FSH and LH during natural ovarian stimulation. Ups J Med Sci 118:153–164
17. Stanton PG, Pozvek G, Burgon PG et al (1993) Isolation and characterization of human LH isoforms. J Endocrinol 138:529–543
18. Burgon PG, Stanton PG, Robertson DM (1996) *In vivo* bioactivities and clearance patterns of highly purified human luteinizing hormone isoforms. Endocrinology 137:4827–4836
19. Yung Y, Aviel-Ronen S, Maman E et al (2014) Localization of luteinizing hormone receptor protein in the human ovary. Mol Hum Reprod 20:844–849
20. Ropelato MG, Garcia-Rudaz MC et al (1999) A preponderance of basic luteinizing (LH) isoforms accompanies inappropriate hypersecretion of both basal and pulsatile LH in adolescents with polycystic ovarian syndrome. J Clin Endocrinol Metab 84:4629–4636
21. Wide L, Eriksson K, Sluss PM, Hull JE (2010) The common genetic variant of luteinizing hormone has a longer half life than the wild type in heterozygous women. J Clin Endocrinol 95:383–389
22. Alviggi C, Petersson K, Longobardi S et al (2013) A common polymorphic allele of the beta-LH subunit gene is associated with higher exogenous FSH consumption during controlled ovarian stimulation for assisted reproductive technology. Reprod Biol Endocrinol 11:51
23. Cole LA (2009) New discoveries on the biology and detection of human chorionic gonadotropin. Reprod Biol Endocrinol 7:1–47
24. Choi J, Smitz J (2014) Luteinizing hormone and human chorionic gonadotropin: distinguishing unique physiologic roles. Gynecol Endocrinol 30:174–181

3 Which Gonadotropin Preparations to Use

The stimulation of ovulation is fundamentally driven by pituitary FSH, the basic hormone for follicular development, with possible assistance from pituitary LH. In clinical practice, ovulation is triggered with placental hCG.

3.1 Follicle-Stimulating Hormone

Four FSH preparations are presently available, each distinguished by its isoform profile. The different profiles result from the hormonal origin and also from the purification process that can significantly affect the composition of the final product. For example, the various hormone purification steps are influenced by the molecular electric charge, yet one can select a less efficient total extraction and purification, or a more efficient process that loses some product [1, 2].

3.1.1 Two Preparations of Human Origin

The two earlier FSH preparations are both extracts of natural hormone from the urine of post-menopausal women.

3.1.1.1 Human Menopausal Gonadotropins or Menotropins (HMG)

HMG is the longest-used preparation, having been developed as a replacement for pregnant mare serum gonadotropins (PMSG) extracted from pregnant horses, used for their FSH effect biologically effective for ovarian stimulation in women. The HMG products *Pergonal*® and *Neopergonal*®, both from Serono, Inc., and *Humegon*® by Organon Co., are all characterized by having a 1:1 ratio of FSH to LH. A second generation of highly purified gonadotropin extract (HP-HMG, (*Menogon*® or *Menopur*®)), was introduced later as an improvement due to several additional purification steps. The LH effect is claimed to be partly related to the pituitary hCG present in the urine, and is important to balance the relative shortage of LH in the

J.-C. Emperaire, *Ovulation Stimulation with Gonadotropins*,
DOI 10.1007/978-3-319-18654-2_3

post-menopausal urine. The existence of hCG secretion by the pituitary is still a matter of debate, and in any case it probably constitutes less than 1 % of the total LH bioactivity of menotropins preparations [Fostimon EU MRP registration, Personal communication to author].

3.1.1.2 Urinary FSH

Urinary FSH (uFSH) first appeared in 1988 as an attempt to eliminate all LH activity that was considered by some to be deleterious for treatment of polycystic ovarian disease (PCOD). To this end FSH was initially concentrated from human post-menopausal urine by using monoclonal antibodies to bind and remove LH. However, this biologically pure FSH (called urofollitropin, trade names *Fertilin*® and *Metrodin*®) was still contaminated by various other urinary proteins. By 1995, FSH was directly isolated from the urine through the use of its own monoclonal antibodies; this highly purified hormone (called uFSH-HP) contained less than 0.1 % LH and less than 5 % of other protein contaminants. In addition, the process enhanced the original hormone concentration of 100–150 IU/mg protein of uFSH to 10,000 IU/mg for uFSH-HP (originally *Metrodin HP*®, presently marketed as *Fostimon*® and *Bravelle*®) [2]. More highly purified FSH contains a higher proportion of the more acidic isoforms, due to characteristics of pituitary FSH secreted after the menopause, and also because less acidic glycoforms are more prone to hepatic metabolism: affinity of the various isoforms for hepatic asialoglycoprotein receptors is diminished in proportion to their sialic acid contents.

Aside from the varied LH content in HMG preparations, there are other contrasts between the available FSH extracts: for example, HMG and uFSH-HP (*Bravelle*®), both manufactured by Ferring Corp, contain lesser amounts of acidic isoforms than does the uFSH-HP (*Fostimon*®) sold by IBSA, SA, because the purification process for the former product was not initially designed to protect the sugar residues of FSH. Purification procedures for *Fostimon*® are able to isolate and preserve glycosylated forms at certain critical steps in the extraction process. This secures a more acidic and more complete mix of FSH isoforms in the final product [Fostimon EU MRP registration, Personal communication to author]. Of the four FSH preparations now available, *Fostimon*® has the most complete isoform profile and the highest proportion of acidic isohormones.

3.1.2 Two Preparations of Synthetic Origin

Two basic synthetic preparations are available, plus two others which despite small variations have the same isoform profiles.

3.1.2.1 Recombinant FSH (rFSH)

Recombinant FSH is manufactured by a genetic engineering process utilizing cells from the Chinese hamster ovary (CHO). These cells are uniquely able to link the two synthesized heterodimers with glycosylation. rFSH introduction in 1997 eliminated the burden of post-menopausal urine collections, and it provided a highly stable injectable solution designed for patient self-administration with a convenient subcutaneous injection pen that also reduces wastage.

In contrast to an rFSH produced in human embryonic kidney (HEK-293) cell lines, the CHO gonadotropin contains less acidic isoform than its extracted counterparts because the process of glycosylation is somewhat less effective in CHO cells than in pituitary gonadotrophs. As a result, commercial rFSH contains less complex carbohydrate, a higher proportion of simple oligosaccharides, no bisecting residue branching, and a tri-sialylated FSH form not found in natural human FSH [3, 4]. Further, because the glycosylation and the purification procedures are somewhat different, the two rFSH products (follitropin alpha, *Gonal F®* and follitropin beta, *Puregon®*) demonstrate distinct isoform profiles. Because follitropin alpha is more acidic [5], its half-life after multiple subcutaneous injections is longer than for follitropin beta (36 h vs 24 h) [6].

Four gonadotropin preparations with FSH effect are actually available for clinical use (Table 3.1). Two additional arrivals to the FSH marketplace provide some interesting issues but do not create new FSH isoform profiles.

The combination of follitropin alpha with lutropin alpha (*Pergoveris®*), available since 2007, modernizes the HMG concept with a 2/1 ratio of FSH/LH. However the FSH isoform profile remains similar to that of follitropin alpha. The 2/1 FSH/LH ratio seems to be especially useful for treatment of hypogonadotropic hypogonadism as well as for multifollicular stimulation. Nevertheless, its FSH isoform profile remains the same as *Gonal F®*.

A long acting rFSH (corifollitropin alpha, *Elonva®*), which combines the beta subunit of follitropin beta with the bulky carboxyl terminal peptide of the beta hCG subunit, has a prolonged presence in plasma as a result of its reduced hepatic and renal elimination. The plasma half-life of this "hybrid FSH" is two to three times longer than that of the usual rFSH, but its isoform profile remains nevertheless the same as for follitropin beta. Following an injection of corifollitropin alpha, the maximal concentration of FSH activity is reached within 2 days, instead of the 4–5 days necessary to obtain the equilibrium concentration with daily injections of rFSH (Fig. 3.1) [7]. Maximum plasma levels are dose-related, and contrasts with the duration of its effect, which remains unaltered at all doses. A single administration of corifollitropin alpha is effective over 7 days, which reduces the number of injections and improves patient comfort. A single dose of corifollitropin alpha has been shown

Table 3.1 Isoform distribution of available FSH preparations (except for HMG because of its LH activity)

Number of terminal sialic acid radical(s)	0 (%)	1 (%)	2 (%)	3 (%)	4 (%)
Fostimon	2	5	36	41	16
Bravelle	<5	2	57	36	<5
Puregon	13	43	33	9	2
Gonal F	8	30	47	12	3
	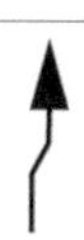	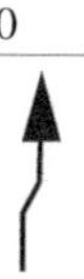			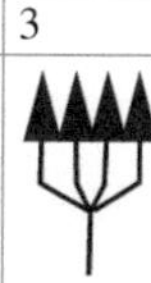

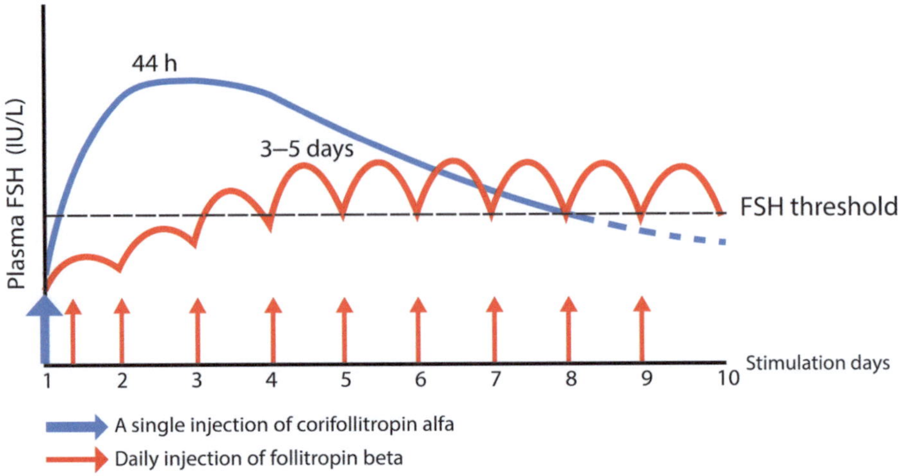

Fig. 3.1 Plasma FSH levels after a single injection of corifollitropin alpha compared with daily injections of rFSH

to have an equal efficacy to daily doses of 200 IU of follitropin beta in normoresponders. On the other hand, the FSH dosage cannot be altered during the single administration period, which makes the ovarian stimulation, and particularly classical stimulations, more challenging [8]. For this reason, use of this long acting FSH product is presently restricted to the initial stimulation phase of an antagonist fixed protocol in the multifollicular stimulation for IVF purposes. Pregnancy rates are comparable to those following the use of daily injections of rFSH [9].

3.1.3 New FSH Preparations To Be Available Soon

3.1.3.1 Human Recombinant FSH

A third rFSH (FE 999049) is being tested by Ferring Pharmaceuticals. Unlike the two others, this recombinant gonadotropin is expressed from a cell line of human fetal retinal origin instead of Chinese hamster ovaries [10].

3.1.3.2 FSH Biosimilar

As a result of patent expiration of recombinant follitropin alpha in most European countries in 2012, the path was opened for a biosimilar recombinant product, with the aim of marketing an effective preparation at lower cost that should permit more couples to gain access to assisted reproduction. Unlike typical generic drugs that are exact reproductions of small synthetic molecules and require only limited comparative data before marketing, this biosimilar material is similar but not identical to the genuine rFSH molecule. rFSH is a large, complex mixture of isoforms that brings a certain degree of microheterogeneity to product activity and safety consequences.

Because the methodological approach to manufacturing follitropin alpha remains cloaked by industrial secrecy, it is not possible to apply the same procedures for use, nor to synthesize an identical biological compound. Recombinant technology for producing rFSH uses eukaryotic cells because they are able to perform the natural and highly important steps of glycosylation and protein folding necessary for the adequate post-translational changes. Different cell strains, each equipped with different glycosylation machinery, produce isoform mixtures of varying activity related to different amounts of heterogeneity. Variations may be further exaggerated by other differences in the extraction, purification, and filling process [11].

At present, international agreements among European nations and the USA have yielded policies for evaluating and approving biosimilar products before their commercialization; other countries, e.g., India, China, and in Latin America, have yet to join. The new guidelines encompass both the pharmacological as well as clinical aspects. However, evaluation of the latter to date is based on only a single prospective study comparing the biosimilar FSH to alpha follitropin, using the number of collected oocytes as the primary endpoint. Alternative endpoints include ongoing pregnancy rates for at least 10 weeks after embryo transfer. Regulations specify that when a biosimilar preparation is approved for one of the indicated uses of alpha follitropin, approval becomes extended for all other indications without need for additional clinical studies.

At this time, marketing of two biosimilar follitropin alpha products has been approved by the European Medicines Agency (EMA):

- *Ovaleap*® (Teva Pharma) is supplied in cartridges "filled by mass" for subcutaneous auto-injections. Results are comparable to *Gonal F*® regarding the average number of collected oocytes, the pregnancy rates in normo-responsive patients, and the rate of ovarian hyperstimulation [12].
- *Bemfola*® (Finox Biotech) is also supplied in prefilled disposable pens for subcutaneous auto-injections. It was shown to be comparable to *Gonal F*® for pharmacokinetic and safety profiles, the average number of collected oocytes as well as for the rate of ovarian hyperstimulation [13, 14].

Whereas biosimilar hormones are expected to be "not inferior" to follitropin alpha, their main impact on cost, outcomes, and safety of assisted reproductive technologies is far from being established. Current information is scarce and derived mainly from studies conducted in individual settings. Further clinical trials will be necessary to develop a better evaluation of effectiveness and safety, especially concerning the risks for ovarian hyperstimulation and immunological side effects [11].

Despite a large number of studies – prospective, retrospective, or meta-analysis – and often with conflicting conclusions, none of the gonadotropin preparations appears on the whole superior to the others, regarding FSH-like effects [15]. For instance, one might think that the synthetic preparations should definitely avoid batch-to-batch inconsistencies, but in fact the extracted urinary preparations show the same consistency, perhaps due to large-sized urine collections and advanced purification procedures. Moreover, the supposedly more sophisticated process of "filling by mass" rather than by biological unitage still fails to obviate variations of bioactivity, even when dosing with identical amounts of measured protein [16]. On the other hand, the "fountain pen" method of administering recombinant preparations facilitates the fractionation of injected doses and minimizes the risk of wasting an expansive medication that so often happens when using vials that require reconstitution of a lyophilized preparation.

3.1.4 Consideration of Therapeutic Goals

As one begins to decide treatment strategy, it is essential to consider the unique isoform profiles of each gonadotropin preparation.

3.1.4.1 Acknowledgment of an FSH Ceiling

Research using isolated intact ovarian follicles has clearly identified an untoward effect of FSH that occurs at levels above a certain hormone concentration. This effect most likely explains many of the disappointing clinical results when high FSH doses are administered during IVF cycles [17]. When high doses appear necessary in certain low-responding patients, it would be most appropriate to choose the more acidic urine-extracted preparations that offer a higher "ceiling," and which seem to minimize the damaging effects upon the follicle and its contents.

3.1.4.2 Anticipating the Ovarian Response to FSH

Because each patient has a somewhat unique isoform profile of her own pituitary FSH, it is important to consider whether this peculiarity might help avoid a poor ovarian response through choosing a more appropriate FSH preparation. Investigations of this concept in the current literature appear to conflict and it may be some time before it is possible to adjust appropriately the nature and the starting doses of FSH in accordance with a patient's own isohormone profile [18, 19].

3.1.4.3 Switching Gonadotropin Preparations

Basically, there are two approaches for deciding to change from one gonadotropin preparation to another.

1. Changing to a different stimulation cycle. Two alternating points of view must be taken into account:
    - Because the isoform profiles of gonadotropins differ in the degree of sialylation, one may expect that each of the four available preparations has a variable therapeutic effect in a given patient, although too subtle to be detected through our monitoring instruments.
    - The unique physiologic qualities of each patient must also be kept in mind. Each has a unique isoform profile for her own secreted gonadotropin, her own pre-ovulatory surge profile, as well as her singular response to a short-lived GnRH agonist. Each patient also has a unique population of ovarian FSH receptors, most certainly adapted to her own isohormone profile. She is likely to respond differently to each gonadotropin preparation.

This makes for a complex situation because a given patient may respond differently to the various available preparations, yet different patients may also show different responses to the same preparation. These variations are well outside the possible monitoring controls, but can result in an exaggerated or dampened FSH response.
The question remains: is it reasonable to use the same FSH preparation for several IVF cycles in each patient? Until the time when pharmaco-genomic analysis identifies the optimal isoform profile match for each patient, we may find it necessary to settle for changing choices of preparations throughout the therapeutic strategy [20].

2. Changing within the same stimulation cycle. Another approach when selecting gonadotropin preparations could be to choose the FSH isoform profiles that most closely mimic the hormones secreted during a normal menstrual cycle, i.e., begin stimulation with a more acidic preparation, and then shift to a less acidic preparation during the immediate pre-ovulatory period [21]. Some studies have indeed demonstrated that this strategy of sequential adjustment results in excellent oocyte quality and good clinical results for IVF procedures [22, 23], and perhaps especially in older patients [24].

3.2 Luteinizing Hormone

Although LH provides an important physiological role in the development of the dominant follicle from the mid-follicular phase forward, it plays a central role in ovarian steroidogenesis. The requisite amounts of this hormone for ovulation stimulation are so low that the process can be induced by exclusive use of FSH preparations. LH must be added to FSH only when endogenous levels of the former fall below 1.2 IU/l, necessary for harmonious follicular growth. This situation is typically found among hypothalamic-pituitary hypogonadotropic anovulatory patients, as well as in some multifollicular stimulations that are co-treated with GnRH agonists.

The only available exclusive LH preparation for therapeutic use is a recombinant hormone product (rLH, luteotropin alpha, *Luveris®*), produced by genetic engineering, and in clinical use since 2000. LH is also available in combinations with FSH:

- Urinary FSH and LH at a 1/1 ratio, as HMG (*Menopur®*)
- Recombinant FSH and LH at a 2/1 ratio (*Pergoveris®*)

The complexity of LH isoforms is comparable to that of FSH. Similarly, each patient has a unique LH glycoform profile. Possible clinical differences in responses to natural LH and rLH might be more difficult to observe, because LH use is so limited and strategic use is often empirical.

3.3 Human Chorionic Gonadotropin

As with other gonadotropins, the hCG preparations that are used for triggering ovulation at the end of the follicular stimulation are derived from two different sources.

Urinary hCG: Very large amounts of bioactive hCG are found in the urine of pregnant women, having been secreted initially by the embryonic pouch, and later by the placenta. Despite several purification steps, the urinary hCG available for clinical use (*Choragon*®, Chorionic Gonadotropins 500, 1,500 and 5,000 IU) still includes most of the 15 different hCG proteins normally present in pregnant urine, including the beta core fragments and residual urinary proteins having no bioactivity. One additional purification step results in a highly purified urinary hCG (uhCG-HP) that is free of residual urinary proteins and which is suitable for sc administration [25].

Recombinant hCG: This most recent of all gonadotropins synthesized by recombinant technology has been available since 2001. rhCG (*Ovidrel*®) is far more pure than uhCG, because it is exclusively composed of the main hCG heterodimer. It includes none of the naturally occurring hCG molecules such as hypersialylated hCG or the free beta subunit, which do have slight biological activity. rhCG preparations have much greater batch-to-batch consistency, and are sold as 250 μg doses expressing a total biological potency between 5,000 and 10,000 IU uhCG. "Fountain pen" syringes are available containing 6,000–6,500 IU that permit precise dosing on a measured scale of 10 μg (50–60 IU).

Despite a number of characteristic distinctions, no differences between the two hCG preparations have been reported with clinical use. However, their endometrial actions do appear somewhat distinct [26, 27].

3.4 Summary and Conclusions

From a practical standpoint, no one preparation of FSH gonadotropins is superior to any of the others. Nonetheless, it is very possible that one preparation may be best suited for *a particular patient*. A clinician's choices are often subjectively decided, and may not be determined solely by a scientific argument. That said, good clinical practice should include frequent re-evaluation of one's choices, whether or not the field provides scientific evidence at the moment. The only certitude is the necessity to add LH to FSH when the former is required for a maximal follicular maturation, such as in the hypothalamic-pituitary hypogonadotropic patient, either as HMG (1/1 ratio) or as *Pergoveris*® (2/1 ratio), or by the addition of suitable amounts of *Luveris*® to FSH in order to adjust to the required ratio.

References

1. Gordon K (2002) New developments in gonadotropin pharmacology. Reprod Biomed Online 5:259–265
2. The Practice Committee of the American Society for Reproductive Medicine (2008) Gonadotropin preparations: past, present, and future. Fertil Steril 90(Suppl 5):S13–S20

3. Ulloa-Aguirre A, Timossi C (1998) Structure and function relationships of follicle-stimulating hormone and its receptor. Hum Reprod Update 4:260–283
4. Harris SD, Anobile CJ, McLoughlin JD et al (1996) Internal carbohydrate complexity of the oligosaccharide chains of recombinant human follicle stimulating hormone (Puregon, Org 32489); a comparison with Metrodin and Metrodin-HP. Hum Reprod 2:371–382
5. Olijve W, DeBoer W, Mulders JW, Wezenbeck PM (1996) Molecular biology and biochemistry of human recombinant follicle stimulating hormone (Puregon). Mol Hum Reprod 2:371–382
6. Follitropins: drug information. Copyright 1978–2006 Lexi-Comp in Up-to date on line version 14.3
7. Corifollitropin alfa Ensure Study Group (2010) Corifollitropin alfa for ovarian stimulation in IVF: a randomized trial in lower-body-weight women. Reprod Biomed Online 21:66–76
8. Rombauts L, Talmor A (2012) Corifollitropin alfa for female infertility. Expert Opin Biol Ther 12:107–112
9. Devroey P, Boostanfar R, Koper NP et al (2009) A double blind, non inferiority RCT comparing corifollitropin alfa and recombinant FSH during the first seven days of ovarian stimulation using a GnRH antagonist protocol. Hum Reprod 12:3063–3072
10. Arce JC, Nyboe C, Andersen A, Fernandez-Sanchez M et al (2014) Relation between dose of FE 999049, a recombinant FSH derived from a human cell line, used for controlled ovarian stimulation, and number of oocytes, embryos and blastocysts. Abstract P-492 of the 30th Annual Meeting of ESHRE, Munich, Germany
11. Santi D, Simoni M (2014) Biosimilar recombinant follicle stimulating hormones in infertility treatment. Expert Opin Biol Ther 14:1399–1409
12. European Medicine Agency (2013) EPAR summary for the public: Ovaleap (follitropin alfa). EMA/562331/2013. Available online
13. European Medicine Agency (2012) EPAR summary for the public: Bemfola (follitropin alfa). EMA /688155/2012. Available online
14. Woltz M, Gouya G, Sator M et al (2015) Comparison of pharmacokinetic and safety profiles between Bemfola® and Gonal-f® after subcutaneous application. Eur J Drug Metab Pharmacokinet, 2015 Jan 30. [Epub ahead of print] PMID: 25633239
15. AFSSAPS (2007) Les médicaments inducteurs de l'ovulation: les gonadotrophines. Argumentaire et Recommandations. Actualisation
16. Wolfenson C, Groisman J, Coulto AS et al (2005) Batch-to-batch consistency of human derived gonadotrophin preparations compared with recombinant preparations. Reprod Med Online 4:442–454
17. Pal L, Jindal S, Witt BR, Santoro N (2009) Less is more: increased gonadotropin use for ovarian stimulation adversely influences clinical pregnancy and live birth after in vitro fertilization. Fertil Steril 89:1694–1701
18. Smeenk JMJ, Braat DDM, Kremer JAM et al (2006) Follicle stimulating hormone isoforms are not useful as pretreatment predictors of outcome in *in vitro* fertilization: a pilot study. Fertil Steril 85:1694–1701
19. Letterie GS, Lee JS, Padmanabhan V (2006) Assessment of ovarian reserve by using the follicle stimulating hormone isoform distribution pattern to predict the outcome of *in vitro* fertilization. Fertil Steril 86:1547–1548
20. Emperaire JC (2009) Savoir changer de gonadotrophine. Gynecol Obstet Fertil 37:291–293
21. Andersen CY (2004) FSH isoform composition of commercial gonadotropin preparations: a neglected aspect? Reprod Biomed Online 9:231–236
22. Pacchiarotti A, Aragona C, Gaglione R, Selman H (2007) Efficacy of a combined protocol of urinary and recombinant follicle stimulating hormone used for ovarian stimulation of patients undergoing ICSI cycles. J Assist Reprod Genet 9:400–405
23. Selman H, Pacchiarotti A, El-Danasouri I (2010) Ovarian stimulation protocols based on follicle stimulating hormone glycosylation pattern: impact on oocyte quality and clinical outcome. Fertil Steril 94:1782–1786

24. Colacurci N, Caprio F, La Verde E et al (2014) Sequential protocol with urinary-FSH/recombinant-FSH versus standard protocol with recombinant-FSH in women of advanced age undergoing IVF. Gynecol Endocrinol 30:730–733
25. Bellavia M, DeGeyter C, Streuli I et al (2013) Randomized control trial comparing highly purified (HP-hCG) and recombinant (rhCG) hCG for triggering ovulation in ART. Gynecol Endocrinol 29:93–97
26. Al Inany H, Alboughar MA, Mansour RT, Proctor M (2005) Recombinant versus urinary gonadotrophins for triggering ovulation in assisted conception. Human Reprod 20:2061–2073
27. Pakanikolaou EG, Bourgain C, Fatemi H et al (2012) Endometrial advancement after triggering with recombinant or urinary HCG: a randomized controlled pilot study. Reprod Endocrinol 21:50–55

In Preparation for the Stimulation 4

The ovary is hardly an isolated organ. It is not only unique to each patient; it is subject to numerous intrinsic and extrinsic factors of the patient's health and disease, as well as to personal and psychosocial environments.

4.1 Searching for Other Hypofertility Factors

Ovulatory stimulation using gonadotropins is a powerful treatment, to be initiated only with sage advice. A complete and thorough preliminary assessment is mandatory to identify and eliminate other factors that may be impeding a couple's fertility or the efficacy of a treatment plan.

A proper evaluation must include:

- A clear hysterosalpingogram, to appraise utero-adnexal integrity. If patency of one or both tubes remains doubtful, a selective salpingogram should be performed. Should the procedure be technically impossible, or if a tubal obstruction is confirmed. Direct visualization also affords the opportunity to search for abnormalities such as adhesions or parietal endometriosis that may be missed by ultrasound scanning. When the integrity of the uterine cavity is doubtful, hysterosonography will confirm or eliminate the need for a hysteroscopy.
- An evaluation of the male partner's fertility based upon a spermiogram and, when possible, supplemented by a post-coital test with spontaneous or estrogen-treated cervical mucus.

It bears noting that discovery of some abnormal findings during these initial explorations does not necessarily obviate ovulation stimulation, but it nevertheless suggests that some additional issues should be considered when developing a therapeutic strategy. Correction of a secondary problem may improve chances for clinical success.

J.-C. Emperaire, *Ovulation Stimulation with Gonadotropins*,
DOI 10.1007/978-3-319-18654-2_4

4.2 Evaluation of the Patient

A patient's age and body mass index (BMI) are certainly two of the more obvious characteristics relevant to success of ovulation induction. However, one must take into account a variety of related malfunctions or ongoing medical treatments.

4.2.1 Patient Age

A relatively advanced age should not automatically eliminate every candidate for ovarian stimulation, provided that FSH levels are not continually elevated. To be sure, numerous experimental studies of donor insemination and IVF have documented the progressive decline of pregnancy rates past the age of 38, even with a satisfactory process of ovulation induction, so age must always be a consideration. There are no reported studies of variations of the FSH threshold in relation to age, but a diminished ovarian response does appear more frequently in the late 30s and beyond, and higher FSH doses are typically needed with older patients. In addition, a substantial variation of individual responses to dosage may be encountered among older patients.

Advancing age does not necessarily alter the prognosis for a successful pregnancy in many types of anovulation. Indeed, time may actually become an ally in the patient of polycystic ovary syndrome. Pregnancy success rates with gonadotropin treatment actually increase in PCOS patients past the age of 36, possibly because of an age-related decrease in the size of the pre-antral follicular cohort.

4.2.2 Patient Weight

Ovulation stimulation should ideally be undertaken in patients within a normal BMI range of 20–25. Deviation from normal brings a variety of problems for a successful stimulation.

4.2.2.1 Insufficient Weight

Weight insufficiency usually occurs in a context of eating disorders that are associated with psychosocial problems. Decisions for stimulating ovulation in these cases should be taken judiciously, inasmuch as achieving a normal weight does not always restore spontaneous menstrual cycling. Ovarian stimulation can be a perplexing task in these low-weight patients because safety margins are narrower. Ovarian responses are somewhat more difficult to anticipate and stimulation should be attempted only when weight and psychological status are believed to have stabilized. Concurrence of a mental health professional should be obtained.

4.2.2.2 Excess Weight

A high proportion of anovulatory women present with weight excess. It is well established that the ovarian response to administered gonadotropins is blunted even when obesity is moderate (BMI<28), perhaps due to a "depot" effect at the injection site in fat-infiltrated tissues combined with an increased volume of distribution. This would explain why increased dosing of gonadotropins, and/or prolonged duration of stimulation, is often necessary in the more obese patient, even when using the IM route: Bioavailability of injected FSH has been shown to be lower in these patients after SC administration than after IM injection [1]. For the same reasons, gonadotropins should be administered just above the knee when the SC route is chosen.

Spontaneous fertility is also lower in the more obese patient, and the risks for miscarriage and perinatal morbidity are higher. There is emerging evidence that leptin, a protein secreted by adipocytes, plays a key role in fertility, and elevated plasma levels are thought to disrupt folliculogenesis, steroid hormone secretion, and endometrial receptivity [2]. Although the overall success rates of obese patients are similar to those of normal weight women, at least in IVF trials, it remains important to attempt significant weight reduction prior to stimulation, using dietary or behavioral modification [3]. Indeed a weight loss of only 2–5 % has been reported sufficient for restoration of spontaneous ovulation within a few months in nearly half of anovulatory overweight patients [4].

All that said, it may be illusionary to hope for significant and stable weight loss in patients with a prolonged history of repeated weight losses and gains. Such a pattern frequently correlates with shifting phases of active to absent motivation about weight reduction, even when reinforced by an increased desire to become pregnant. Bariatric surgery may be cautiously considered in some instances. Because declining to help a patient with persistent obesity may represent for her yet another failure, it would be well advised to negotiate a "contract" of weight stability. By recording and discussing body weight during each monitoring appointment, one may pose the prospect of interrupting the stimulation protocol until the patient is able to return to a previously agreed weight. It is also important to refute the notion in the mind of heavy patients that "hormones put weight on."

In patients with polycystic ovarian syndrome (PCOS), a peripheral insulin resistance is often encountered that leads to a hyperinsulinemia and an independent risk factor for obesity. Because weight loss, however difficult to achieve, may be necessary before embarking on ovarian stimulation, it may be advantageous to add metformin together with the stimulation itself [5]. Even if an obese patient succeeds in becoming pregnant, her excess weight adds additional risk to the pregnancy that is usually correlated with the degree of weight excess. Hypertension, diabetes, and perinatal complications can turn this apparent success into a very dismal outcome. Ovulation stimulation must be careful to avoid unreasonable and risky procedures.

4.2.2.3 Associated Pathologies

The prospect of ovarian stimulation and pregnancy provides a very appropriate time to heighten a patient's awareness of the deleterious effects of alcohol, tobacco, and numerous other toxic substances on oocyte reserve and quality. It is also important to take into account a number of other associated risk factors before beginning the treatment:

- *Chronic diseases*: If one can establish that a given patient's underlying chronic conditions such as a demyelinating syndrome, colorectal hemorrhage, epilepsy, or cardiovascular complications will likely be compatible with the prospect of a pregnancy, then the syndrome can be anticipated to be similarly compatible with protocols of ovarian stimulation. However, it is important to contact the patient's specialist before beginning therapy in order to uncover potential hazards. For example, it is crucial to avoid all risk, however small it may be, for an ovarian hyperstimulation situation in a patient with an established coagulation disorder. Another example for caution would occur in a patient being treated for systemic lupus erythematosus, because her ovarian reserve may have been compromised even in the absence of alkylating treatment [6].

- *Previous history of (extra-ovarian) cancer*: It is difficult to comprehend why an oncologist would recommend against ovarian stimulation while still consenting to a pregnancy in a patient with a history of cancer. The levels of plasma estradiol resulting from a monofollicular stimulation protocol remain very close to those of the physiologic menstrual cycle. Even with a multifollicular protocol that might be used for IVF, the relatively high estradiol levels found during mid- to late follicular phase of a stimulated cycle are minimal compared to those which will flood a patient during the 9 months of pregnancy. This example of a "precaution principle" needs to be discussed each time with the patient's oncologist in order to agree on the strategy best suited to the patient's condition.
- *Medications*. Each patient's therapies must be carefully evaluated, even if they do not appear as directly detrimental to ovarian stimulation, because it is also highly important to anticipate continued management of therapies once a pregnancy begins. This would be especially true for cytotoxic or psychoactive medications.

4.3 Evaluation of Ovarian Status

A thorough evaluation of the ovarian condition is a fundamental step. One must evaluate the complement of follicles, and thus the potential sensitivity to FSH and prognosis for stimulation. A woman's oocyte reserve decreases steadily from intrauterine life until menopause: from a mean of 100,000 at age 20–30,000 at age 30, and only 8,000 remaining at 40 years of age [7]. Although stem germ cells that appear capable of division and differentiation may be found in the adult female ovary, the reserve of primordial follicles must be considered as finite [8]. The ovarian endowment of oocytes should be assessed around the third day of the cycle (CD 2–5) using both ultrasound and hormonal measures.

4.3.1 Hormonal Parameters

4.3.1.1 FSH

Determination of plasma FSH remains a principal index, because levels increase as the follicular supply decreases. However the correlation between these two variables is far from tight, because FSH levels can fluctuate widely in blood. While a continuously elevated FSH level (>15 IU/l) is probably an early sign of ovarian insufficiency, moderately elevated FSH levels below 15 IU/l indicate only a need for a very cautious interpretation.

FSH secretion is pulsatile with peaks about every 90 min during the follicular phase. Thus a best evaluation of FSH should be performed on three pooled blood samples taken at 20 min intervals, a practice that is not routinely conducted. In addition, the normal range of plasma FSH varies between laboratories and also between hormone assay systems. Upper levels of normal can vary from 9.5 to 12 IU/l in individual laboratories.

While abnormally high FSH levels are usually confirmed by repeated observations in successive cycles, a pattern of normal FSH mixed interspersed with elevated readings should be taken as a warning for a declining ovarian reserve: in these cases, however, overall results from stimulations are not better when started on a cycle with a subnormal FSH value. Some patients with moderately elevated FSH (10–13 IU/l) demonstrate nevertheless a normal ability to achieve pregnancy on stimulation; this could reflect a physiological variation such as an FSH receptor polymorphism. Such a possibility must be kept in mind when working with young patients before considering oocyte donation. An attempt to stimulate follicular growth can still be carried out in these cases, although it may well require higher FSH doses in order to be successful.

On the other hand, levels of plasma FSH do not correlate well with oocyte quality. Fertility prognosis is actually better in women under 35 years of age and with moderately elevated FSH, compared to older women having FSH in the normal range [9]. Toner's formula remains valid: FSH levels are a measure of oocyte quantity, whereas the patient's age remains the best index of oocyte quality [10].

Use of dynamic assessments of FSH through administration of clomiphene or with a GnRH agonist in order to clarify the significance of borderline values are often disappointing, because of the intricacy of both the method and of its interpretation. In the end, the results are no more discriminating than by taking a single basal hormone measurement [11]. Similarly, the "Effort Test," done by measuring estradiol secretion after FSH administration (a revival of the Netter test first described in 1968), is also disappointing [12]. These tests are better replaced by simply conducting an actual attempt to stimulate ovulation.

Estradiol. Isolated measures of estradiol alone are not very accurate markers of ovarian reserve, but are mandatory for the interpretation of the FSH level. Estradiol must be assayed at the same moment as FSH. An early developing ovarian insufficiency may be expressed with high estradiol values on CD 3 (>70 pg/ml) that will decrease and normalize FSH secretion via negative feedback.

Inhibin B. This glycoprotein of the TGF beta family is produced by the granulosa cells under the stimulating effect of FSH. It also inhibits pituitary secretion of FSH through a negative feedback mechanism. Because inhibin B levels move in the opposite direction of FSH, it was originally thought to be a reliable marker of ovarian reserve. However, a number of literature reports have described a fluctuating and poorly discriminating nature, and interest in its use as a marker of follicular reserve integrity has finally diminished.

Anti-Müllerian hormone (AMH). Another glycoprotein of the TGF-β family, AMH is presently considered as the best hormonal marker of ovarian reserve. Like Inhibin B, it is also produced by granulosa cells of primary follicles. Expression is highest in pre-antral and antral follicles, which then undergoes a gradual decline as the follicles mature further. AMH expression is highest in follicles of less than 4 mm in diameter, a size when they become sensitive to FSH, and the hormone serves to inhibit follicular transition from primordial to pre-antral stage. It also decreases the antral follicle sensitivity to FSH.

In contrast to other proposed hormonal markers, AMH secretion remains rather steady throughout the menstrual cycle. Some reports have suggested that levels decrease somewhat throughout the follicular phase and during multifollicular stimulation protocols, as the pre-antral and antral follicles grow larger and gradually cease secreting the hormone [13, 14]. Values are generally reproducible from one cycle to the next [15]. A level greater than 2 ng/ml is usually considered as evidence for a satisfactory ovarian reserve. However reports of substantial heterogeneity of quality of early AMH assay kits threw doubt on the validity of AMH values, and an abnormal value must always be considered with caution. Modified, improved assay procedures seem to have resolved much of the uncertainty at present, but are still lacking of an international standard [16]. AMH levels decline steadily during multifollicular stimulation in correlation with the rise of estradiol levels, confirming that growing follicles cease to secrete AMH [14]. On the other hand, it must be acknowledged that anti-Müllerian hormone has limited discriminative value concerning oocyte quality or regarding prospects for achieving a successful pregnancy [17]. On the other hand, AMH levels may be temporarily depressed by hormonal contraceptives, GnRH agonists, after pelvic surgery or in case of hypogonadotropic hypogonadism [18, 19].

To summarize, interpretation of these various hormonal values when attempting to estimate ovarian reserve, and also for devising treatment strategies for infertile couples, should nevertheless be taken with the benefit of hindsight and a great deal of caution, because they represent only statistical data that may not apply successfully to a particular patient [20]. In Hall's retrospective study, for instance, half of the 78 patients who achieved pregnancy through IVF initially showed abnormally low values of both inhibin B and AMH [21].

4.3.2 Ultrasound Parameters

Ovarian follicle quantity. The technology involved in making antral follicle counts (AFC), usually conducted on the same cycle day that the hormonal measures are made, has been substantially improved with the latest generation of high frequency endovaginal probes that are capable of visualizing follicles as small as 2 mm diameter. Ultrasound now provides a direct view of the follicular cohort, but with some inter-cycle or inter-observer and intra-observer variations. Among the various hormonal parameters, plasma AMH correlates best with AFC as an indicator of the ovarian reserve [22]. Normally, the total AFC of visible structures at least 2 mm diameter is between 15 and 25 for the pair of "normofollicular" ovaries, although the number on each may not be equal. The capacity for an ovarian response to stimulation begins to decrease with AFC totals below 15, and it becomes problematic when fewer than five follicles are visible ("paucifollicular" ovaries) [23]. A higher number of follicles visible on each ovary (e.g., greater than 25) defines "multifollicular" and "micro-polycystic" conditions, and responses to gonadotropins may differ in these situations. Multifollicular ovaries show follicles of varied sizes distributed throughout the whole gonad, whereas the micro-polycystic ovary is characterized by the presence of numerous very small follicles squeezed together inside the ovarian cortex, and usually with a condensed ovarian stroma. These two conditions may be difficult to distinguish with certainty, particularly as the definitions of PCO remain imprecise. According to the most recent consensus conference, the visible follicles count necessary to establish a diagnosis continues to increase as technical sophistication of vaginal probes improves [22]. Three-dimensional ultrasound technology seems to offer little improvement for AFC protocols, which remains satisfactory by 2D imagery. In the end, it is simply the response of ovary itself, whether normal or explosive, to a conventional step up stimulation protocol, that makes the difference.

Follicular size. Measures of follicular size within the AFC are also significantly important, as smaller follicles (<5 mm) show a better predictive value than the larger ones (5–10 mm) [24].

Ovarian volume: Ovarian volume has also been proposed as a marker of ovarian reserve. While relatively easy to perform, this measure appears to provide little superior information than does the standard AFC [25].

4.3.3 Practical Indications for Evaluating Ovarian Reserve

Although assessment of ovarian reserve may not be always necessary, it is always useful prior to beginning treatment of an infertile couple.

Mono- or Paucifollicular Stimulation: A routine preliminary measure of the ovarian reserve markers would not appear to be mandatory for a patient under 35 years of age, unless she has a history of possible ovarian trauma (e.g., pelvic surgery or chemotherapy) or of endometriosis. It may become useful in cases when a younger patient has a poor response to an initial trial, or if a paucifollicular appearance is observed with ultrasound. On the other hand, an occasional young patient may show an already declining ovarian reserve, as this phenomenon is silent and can develop without apparent causes. Thus a growing number of clinicians recommend a routine assay of plasma AMH no matter the age of an infertile patient, and even in non-infertile patients who seek to delay their pregnancy for a later time [26]. Past the age of 35, evaluation of ovarian reserve becomes necessary in order to assess a possible alteration that would change the therapeutic strategy. For this evaluation the best combination is a measure of plasma AMH and the AFC, with measures of plasma FSH adding another prognostic factor when the initial two markers yield low values.

Multifollicular Stimulation. In this case, assessment of ovarian reserve is always necessary, whatever the patient's age, in order to evaluate more precisely the follicular cohort size. This will help to establish a starting dose of gonadotropins and to anticipate the ovarian response. Here, too, AMH and AFC become the best choices, and are closely correlated, as they measure he same follicular pool; however, their performances characteristics are different and they cannot be really considered as interchangeable, AMH being at present the best measure of ovarian reserve and the most reliable predictive parameter of ovarian response [27].

References

1. Dobbs KE, Dumesic JA, Shapiro SS (1994) Differences in serum follicle-stimulating hormone uptake after intramuscular and subcutaneous human menopausal gonadotropin injection. Fertil Steril 62:978–983
2. Pantasri T, Norman RJ (2014) The effects of being overweight and obese on female reproduction: a review. Gynecol Endocrinol 30:90–94
3. Koning AM, Mutsaerts MA, Kuchenbecker WK et al (2012) Complications and outcome of assisted reproductive technologies in overweight and obese women. Hum Reprod 27:457–467
4. Clark AM, Ledger W, Galletly C et al (1995) Weight loss results in significant improvement in pregnancy and ovulation rates in anovulatory obese women. Hum Reprod 10:2705–2712
5. Cheang KI, Nestler JE (2004) Should insulin-sensitizing drugs be used in the treatment of polycystic ovary syndrome? Reprod Biomed Online 8:440–447
6. Wenhong M, Zhongping Z, Xiaoyan L et al (2013) Subclinical impairment of ovarian reserve in systemic lupus erythematous patients with normal menstruation not using alkylating therapy. J Women Health (Larchmt) 22(12):1023–1027
7. Block E (1952) Quantitative morphological investigation of the follicular system in women: variations at different ages. Acta Anat 14:108–123
8. White Y, Woods DC, Yashushi-Takai I et al (2012) Oocyte formation by mitotically active germ cells purified from ovaries of reproductive-age women. Nat Med 18:413–421
9. Luna M, Grunfeld L, Mukherjee T et al (2007) Moderately elevated levels of basal follicle-stimulating hormone in young patients predict low ovarian response, but should not be used to disqualify patients from attempting in vitro fertilization. Fertil Steril 87:782–787
10. Toner JP (2003) Age = egg quality, FSH level = egg quantity. Fertil Steril 79:491
11. Merviel P, Lourdel E, Cabry R et al (2009) L'exploration de la réserve ovarienne dans le bilan d'infertilité. La Lettre du Gynécologue 343:31–36
12. Netter A, Salomon Bernard Y, Millet D (1968) Test de stimulation ovarienne par les HMG. In: Les Gonadotrophines d'Origine Humaine. Byla-Sarle Ed, Paris, pp 31–41
13. Wunder DM, Bersinger NA, Yared DM et al (2008) Statistically significant changes of anti-Müllerian hormone and inhibin levels during the physiologic menstrual cycle in reproductive age women. Fertil Steril 89:927–933
14. Bottcher B, Tsybulyak I, Grubinger T et al (2013) Dynamics of anti-Müllerian hormone during controlled ovarian stimulation. Gynecol Endocrinol 30:121–125
15. Fanchin R, Schonauer LM, Gighini C et al (2003) Serum anti-Mullerian hormone is more strongly related to ovarian follicular status than serum inhibin B, estradiol, FSH and LH on day 3. Hum Reprod 18:323–327
16. Han X, McShane M, Sahertian R et al (2014) Pre-mixing serum samples with assay buffer is a prerequisite for reproducible anti-Müllerian hormone measurement using the Beckman Coulter Gen II assay. Hum Reprod 29:1042–1048

17. Berwanger DA, Silva AL, Even M et al (2010) Hormone antimullerienne: acteur et marqueur de la folliculogènese. Gynecol Obstet Fertil 38:471–474
18. Tanprasertkul C, Manusook S, Somprasit C et al (2014) Antimullerian hormone changes after laparoscopic ovarian cystectomy for endometrioma compared with the nonovarian conditions. Minim Invasive Surg 2014:654856
19. Chan C, Liu K (2014) Clinical pregnancy in a woman with idiopathic hypothalamic hypogonadisme and low AMH: utility of ovarian reserve markers in IHH. J Assist Reprod Genet 31(10):1317–1321
20. Loh JS, Maheshwari A (2011) Anti-Mullerian hormone – is it a crystal ball for predicting ovarian aging? Hum Reprod 26:2925–2932
21. Hall JE, Welt CK, Cramer DW (1999) Inhibin A and inhibin B reflect ovarian function in assisted reproduction but are less useful at predicting outcome. Hum Reprod 14:409–415
22. Dewailly D, Gronier H, Poncelet E et al (2011) Diagnosis of polycystic ovary syndrome (PCOS): revisiting the threshold values of follicle count on ultrasound and the serum AMH levels for the definition of polycystic ovaries. Hum Reprod 26:3123–3129
23. Muttukrishna S, Mc Garrigle H, Wakim R et al (2005) Antral follicle count, anti-Müllerian hormone, and inhibin B: predictors of ovarian response in assisted reproductive technology? BJOG 112:1384–1390
24. Klinkert ER, Broekmans F, Looman CV et al (2005) The antral count is a better marker than basal follicle-stimulating hormone for the selection of older patients with acceptable pregnancy prospects after *in vitro* fertilization. Fertil Steril 83:811–814
25. Syrop CH, Dawson JD, Husman KJ et al (1999) Ovarian volume may predict assisted reproductive outcomes better than follicle stimulating hormone concentration on day 3. Hum Reprod 14:1752–1756
26. Tremellen K, Savulescu J (2014) Ovarian reserve screening: a scientific and ethical analysis. Hum Reprod 29:2606–2614
27. Illiodromiti S, Anderson RA, Nelson SM (2014) Technical and performance characteristics of anti-Müllerian hormone and antral follicle count as bio- markers of ovarian response. Hum Reprod Update. Epub on 11 June 2015

5 Monotoring Ovarian Stimulation

A proper evaluation of the stimulation process includes both functional (i.e., hormonal measures) and morphological (i.e., ultrasound visualization) indices. The combined evaluation should identify a comfort zone between inadequate and excessive stimulation. Zone parameters are assuredly different for mono- or paucifollicular (classic) stimulations on the one hand, and multifollicular (for IVF) stimulations on the other.

5.1 Hormonal (Functional) Monitoring

The only essential hormonal parameter is the rapid plasma estradiol assay, but the evaluation process may be strengthened by addition of LH and/or progesterone measures.

5.1.1 Estradiol

Estradiol assumes the role of lead indicator because its level in blood reflects secretory activity of the dominant ovarian follicle coupled with that of numerous smaller follicles that have developed directly in response to the injected gonadotropins. For this reason pre-ovulatory estradiol is normally higher in stimulated cycles than in the spontaneous cycle. In the natural cycle, the dominant follicle releases estradiol in regularly increasing amounts from the sixth day CD until the pre-ovulatory peak, usually in the range of 125–250 pg/ml.

5.1.2 Progesterone

Measuring progesterone concomitantly with estradiol is a valuable safeguard because it represents another marker of the stimulation quality. However, levels should remain under 1 ng/ml throughout the stimulation process and readings that exceed 1 ng/ml would likely suggest one of the following:

J.-C. Emperaire, *Ovulation Stimulation with Gonadotropins*,
DOI 10.1007/978-3-319-18654-2_5

- An unnoticed ovulation that occurred between two monitoring controls
- An abnormally developing stimulation, despite the presence of satisfactory estradiol and ultrasound parameters
- An inappropriately early follicular luteinization caused by erratic surges of endogenous pituitary LH
- The release of progesterone into blood as a result of FSH-promoted secretion from granulosa cells

During a normal follicular phase, progesterone originates in the theca interna and is converted to androgens for transport to granulosa cells where the production of estradiol is completed. In case of a relative lack of LH, more of the progesterone production may enter the blood instead of being moved along the steroidogenic pathways. An inappropriate increase of blood progesterone results in a thickened cervical mucus and an abnormally matured uterine endometrium that becomes visible on ultrasound. The stimulation cycle should be stopped when this occurs, although the treatment protocol should not necessarily be modified upon the initial occurrence. However, a repeated rise of plasma progesterone during a second consecutive treatment cycle should lead to consideration of protocol modification, or possibly to changing the gonadotropin itself. A progesterone level in excess of 5 ng/ml in the first monitoring sample might be a sign of an early pregnancy. Even if the patient believes she had a normal menses, a pregnancy test would be indicated.

5.1.3 Luteinizing Hormone

A serum LH assay is mandatory when an intra-uterine insemination is planned, but LH measures are also useful for a simple stimulation cycle intended for a single intercourse, in order to know if a spontaneous ovulatory process might have begun prior to hCG administration, a sign of optimal follicular maturity, or if it is the hCG administration that will trigger the ovulation:

An LH rise together with a concomitant progesterone rise suggests that a spontaneous ovulatory process has started within the previous 12–24 h, and that an ovulation will occur on the following day. It will no longer be possible to block this spontaneous event by means of a GnRH antagonist.

An LH rise in excess of twice its initial level, but *without* a progesterone elevation, is an early sign of a spontaneous ovulation that will likely occur 2 days hence; this is similar to the timing that follows an hCG administration. In this situation the spontaneous gonadotropin surge may still be arrested, or at least delayed, if necessary, by using a GnRH antagonist.

5.2 Ultrasound (Morphologic) Monitoring

Ultrasonic imagery for the purpose of monitoring ovulation is best performed though the endo-vaginal route because it places the ultrasound probe in the closest position relative to the pelvic organs being examined. Typical 2D imagery is sufficient to visualize the numbers of growing follicles as well as their shape, location, growth rate, and echogenicity. The images may also help clarify reasons why similar estradiol levels can occur with different types of follicular cohorts. The imagery should also help grade the thickness and echogenicity of the uterine mucosa, as well as the extent of cervical mucus secretion.

5.2.1 Ovarian Follicles

Ovarian follicles appear as transonic structures within the ovary. The mean diameter of a follicle is estimated by the average of two perpendicular diameters, with the calipers placed in contact with the internal follicular wall [1].

In a normal, spontaneous cycle, the selected follicle appears on CD 6 with a diameter of 10 mm, then it expands at a daily rate of 1–2 mm until reaching 15 mm diameter on CD 10. Expansion continues at 2.5 mm daily until ovulation, and may even accelerate during the final hours. A mature follicle typically measures 20–23 mm just prior to rupture [2].

5.2.2 Endometrium

Endometrial appearance and thickness can vary considerably throughout a spontaneous menstrual cycle and also during ovulation stimulation. The thickness of the endometrial mucosa should be measured close to the uterine fundus.

Beginning at the end of menses in a natural menstrual cycle, the follicular phase endometrium grows at a rate of about 1.5 mm daily, reaching a total thickness of 8–10 mm by CD 12. By this time the tissue has developed a 3-layered hypoechogenic ("coffee bean") appearance that changes after ovulation due to the effect of luteal progesterone that arrests further growth (Figs. 5.1 and 5.2) [3].

Recent advances in 3D ultrasound imagery that include automated follicle measurements would seem to be of value only in multifollicular stimulations, where the more numerous follicles have become pressed together. Distorted shapes can

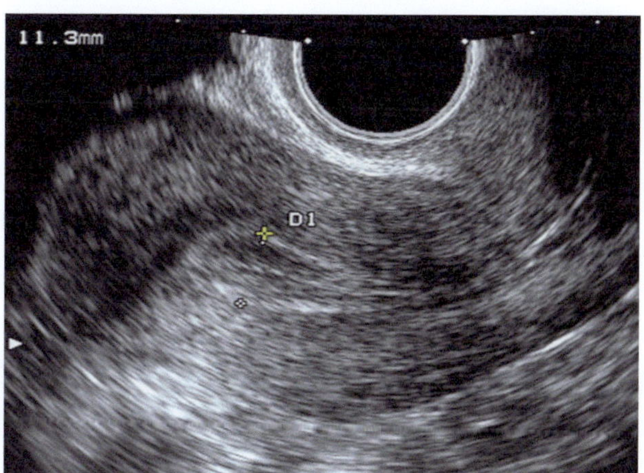

Fig. 5.1 Preovulatory endometrium with three layers showing a characteristic "coffee bean" appearance (Image courtesy of P. Billet)

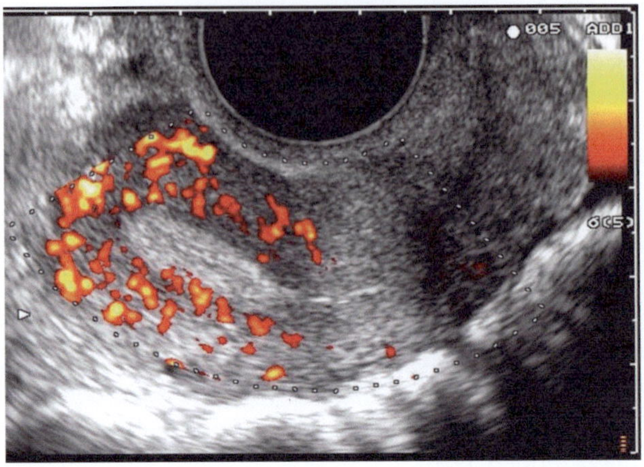

Fig. 5.2 Post-ovulatory echogenic endometrium, with its vascularization visible through color energy Doppler (Image courtesy of P. Billet)

disrupt relations between the mean diameter and the true follicular volume [4]. It remains to be seen whether 3D technology will really improve routine monitoring of classical stimulations.

In order to optimize chances of a good stimulation while avoiding excessive risks, a strategy of evaluating both hormonal and ultrasonic parameters is best. Some studies on exclusively hormonal, or exclusively sonographic, monitoring, or even totally blind stimulation have been published, but they were concerned only with COH, and represented simple feasibility exercises [5]. In the event that the triggering criteria are not met, only the combination of dual hormonal and ultrasound measures provides a complete assessment of the three basic principles that underlie the FSH dosing strategy:

- When estradiol correlates correctly with the follicular diameter(s), the FSH dose should remain unchanged
- When estradiol rises in excess of the follicular growth, the FSH dose should be decreased
- When estradiol lags behind follicular growth, the FSH dosage should be increased, unless a relative LH insufficiency has been detected

Criteria for follicular maturity and ovulation triggering may vary according to the stimulation protocol, and additional discussion of posology will be undertaken in the succeeding chapters.

5.3 Monitoring After hCG Administration

Whereas follicular stimulation typically commands the clinician's close attention, care can easily wane as soon as hCG is administered, almost as if a harmonious progress into the second part of the cycle were obvious. The quality of the luteal gland is of course strictly dependent upon an optimal follicular maturation, but the results of hormonal and ultrasonic monitoring during the pre-ovulatory period can only approximate actual follicle and oocyte maturity. It is well established that hCG administration with an immature or a post-mature follicle will lead to diminished chances for a successful pregnancy.

A normal luteal phase should demonstrate a clear shift of basal body temperature to a higher plateau lasting 12–14 days, and/or a plasma progesterone level in excess of 10 ng/ml on the seventh to ninth post-hCG day. On the other hand, complete follicular rupture does not always occur, and can be confirmed only by ultrasound imagery. Some studies have reported as much as a 40 % incidence of luteinized unruptured follicles (LUF) during stimulated cycles triggered with an hCG injection [6]. Color energy Doppler is now sufficiently sensitive to differentiate the characteristic vascularity of a cystic corpus luteum from an unruptured follicle (Figs. 5.3, 5.4, and 5.5) [7].

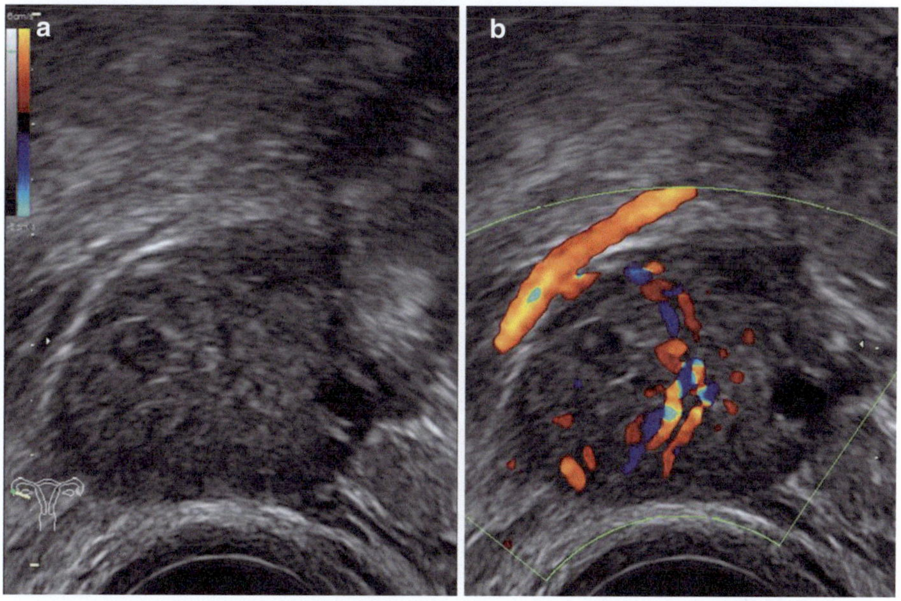

Fig. 5.3 An intra-ovarian corpus luteum that is barely discernible with conventional ultrasound (**a**), but is clearly revealed through color energy Doppler (**b**) (Image courtesy of P. Billet)

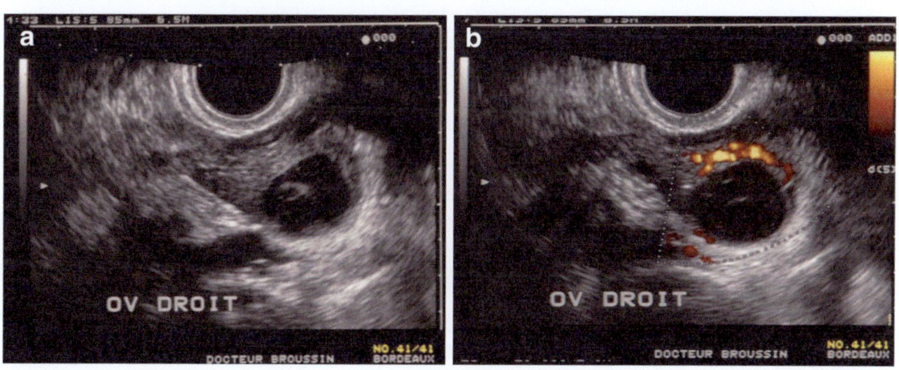

Fig. 5.4 An apparent unruptured follicle 72 h post-hCG seen by conventional ultrasound (**a**) but which is in fact a cystic corpus luteum revealed by color energy Doppler (**b**) (Image courtesy of B. Broussin)

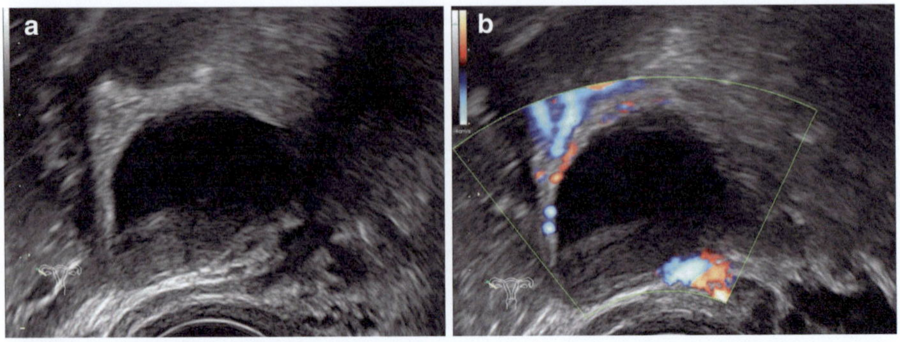

Fig. 5.5 A residual follicle 72 h post-hCG (**a**): color energy Doppler shows an unruptured follicle (**b**) (Image courtesy of P. Billet)

In the latter case, a second administration of hCG may provoke complete follicular rupture and restore chances for a successful pregnancy. An additional sonographic verification on the third post-hCG day is indicated even during the first attempt at a stimulation, and should become a standard procedure if several treated cycles of apparently good quality have not resulted in a pregnancy.

References

1. Duijkers IJ, Louwe LA, Braat DD, Klippig C (2004) One, two or three: how many directions are useful in transvaginal ultrasound measurement of ovarian follicles? Eur J Obstet Gynecol Reprod Biol 117:60–63
2. Bakos O, Lundkvist O, Wide L, Bergh T (1994) Ultrasonographical and hormonal description of the normal ovulatory menstrual cycle. Acta Obstet Gynecol Scand 73:790–796
3. Broussin B (2007) The clinical value of ultrasound for endometrial receptivity assessment in Assisted Reproductive Techniques (ART) procedures. Gynecol Obstet Fertil 35:570–615
4. Salama S, Torre A, Paillusson B et al (2011) La monitorage de l'ovulation: passe, présent et perspectives. Gynecol Obstet Fertil 39:245–254
5. Wiser A, Gonen O, Ghetler Y et al (2012) Monitoring stimulated cycles during *in vitro* fertilization treatment with ultrasound only – preliminary results. Gynecol Endocrinol 28:429–431
6. Check JH, Nazari A, Barnea ER et al (1993) The efficiency of short-term gonadotropin releasing hormone agonists versus human chorionic gonadotropin to enable oocyte release in gonadotropin stimulated cycles. Hum Reprod 8:568–571
7. Miyazaki T, Tanaka M, Miyakoshi K et al (1998) Power and colour Doppler ultrasonography for the evaluation of the vasculature of the human corpus luteum. Hum Reprod 13:2836–2841

6 Triggering Ovulation

Ovulation is simply the focal destruction of the follicular wall that enables extrusion of the oocyte and follicular contents through the breach. A space of some 36–40 h passes from the initial gonadotropin surge to the follicular rupture itself, during which irreversible actions reprogram the entire structure and function of the follicle, reawaken oocyte meiosis, alter the follicular wall, and commence the process of luteinization.

6.1 The Ovulatory Process

6.1.1 Oocyte Maturation

The surge of pituitary gonadotropins provokes a resumption of meiosis in the oocyte nucleus that had been suspended in prophase of the first meiotic division since intrauterine life. As the first polar body is expelled, meiosis arrests once more in metaphase of the second meiotic division, and will be completed only after the ovum is fertilized. Oocyte cytoplasmic maturation develops in the same way, being marked by characteristic granulations that migrate under the cell's cortical membrane.

6.1.2 Follicular Rupture

This event terminates a process of biochemical transformations that result in an increased internal pressure and a weakened follicular wall. The gonadotropin surge inhibits further synthesis of basal membrane components and stimulates proteolytic enzymes, both of which contribute to a weakening of the follicular wall. Gonadotropins also induce an enzymatic deterioration of large follicular fluid proteins into numerous smaller molecules, a process that augments osmotic pressure and a diffusion of water into the follicle. The combination of follicular swelling acting on a weakened wall leads to a rupture that completes the ovulation [1]. This

J.-C. Emperaire, *Ovulation Stimulation with Gonadotropins*,
DOI 10.1007/978-3-319-18654-2_6

stepwise chain of events occurring within the follicle explains the latency period between the start of the pre-ovulatory gonadotropin surge and the completed rupture. It also helps understand why a defective component of this process may lead to an unruptured follicle (luteinized unruptured follicle, LUF syndrome).

Follicular luteinization actually commences just before oocyte extrusion, although theca interna vascularity invades the previously avascular granulosa layer only after ovulation. The luteal body, or corpus luteum, continues to secrete a reduced level of estradiol for a few days because of the perturbations of follicular rupture, and then pre-ovulatory levels return only to decline again at the end of the cycle. Primarily the new luteal gland secretes high levels of progesterone (>10 ng/ml in plasma) before declining as well at the end of the luteal phase. Corpus luteum waning is an apoptotic process programmed to start after 12–14 days, unless the gland has been rescued by exponentially rising secretions of hCG from an implanting embryo.

6.2 Spontaneous Triggering of Ovulation

Natural ovulation is triggered by a pre-ovulatory surge of both pituitary gonadotropins FSH and LH, secondary to a rise of GnRH secretion into the hypothalamic-pituitary portal system (Fig. 6.1).

6.2.1 The Normal Menstrual Cycle

Wave profiles of LH secretion have been analyzed in some detail. Typical pre-ovulatory surges, lasting about 48 h, begin with an ascending phase of 14 h, settle at a plateau for another 10 h, and move through a 24 h declining phase [2]. Although a few cycle-to-cycle variations are possible, each woman seems to have a fairly unique pre-ovulatory surge profile [3]. Profiles can be substantially different between women, particularly with regard to two important parameters (Fig. 6.2):

- *Magnitude*: Surge levels in blood can vary between 25 and 150 IU/l in different individuals, and the intensity seems to correlate with the chance of achieving pregnancy within that cycle.
- *Duration*: Often consistent with the surge magnitude, duration correlates even better with the chance of the cycle ending in a pregnancy [4].

The physiologic importance of the synchronous FSH surge, while of a lesser magnitude (5–12 IU/l) than LH, is less completely established, but it is well understood that FSH plays an important role in the follicular expansion leading to ovulation. In fact, it is possible to trigger an ovulation (or at least the resumption of meiosis) in controlled ovarian hyperstimulation (COH) with FSH alone [5]. It has also been claimed that addition of an FSH bolus to the ovulation-triggering hCG administration results in a superior quality of oocyte and embryo [6]. It is probable that the two gonadotropins act in synergy during the pre-ovulatory surge, and concurrently optimize the ovulatory process and development of the corpus luteum.

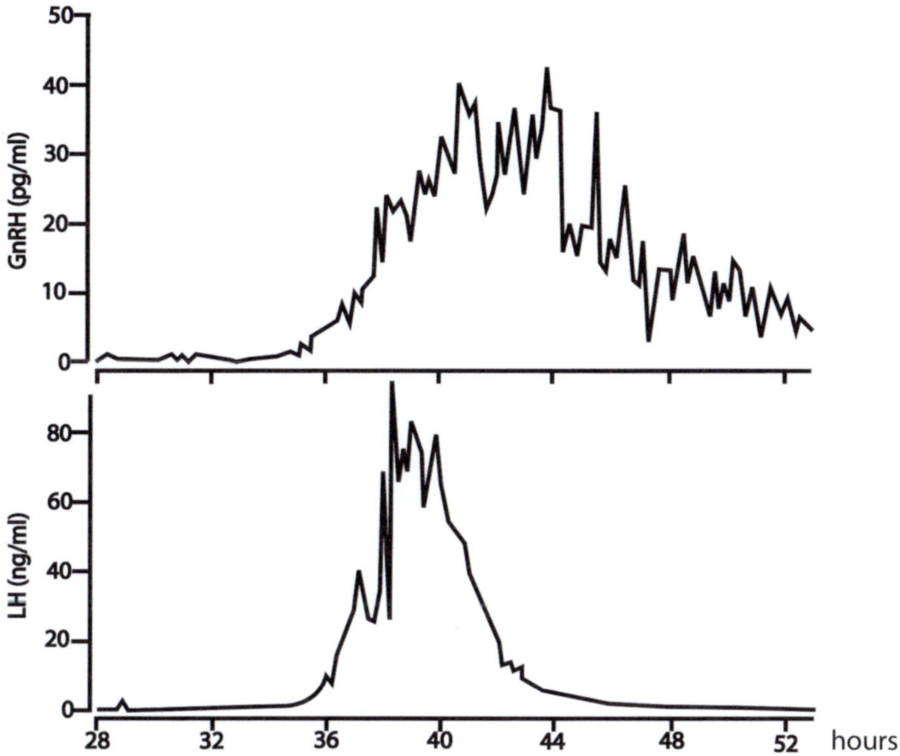

Fig. 6.1 GnRH and gonadotropin pre-ovulatory surges. Note the secondary pituitary desensitization provoked by sustained secretion of GnRH [35]

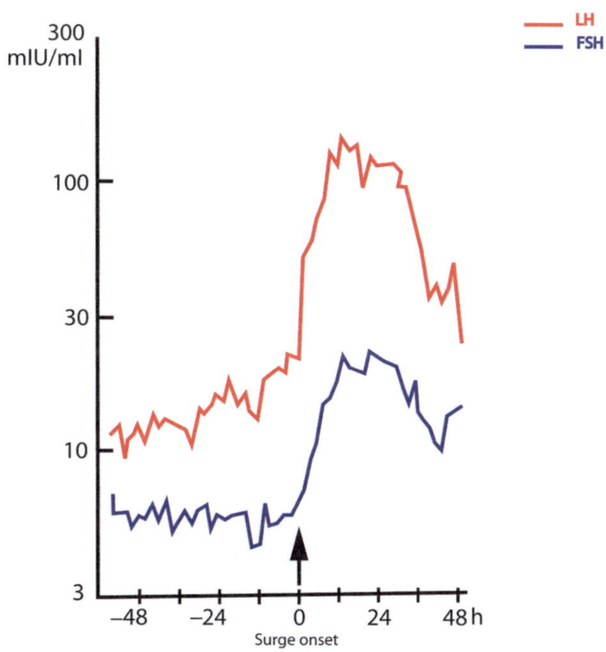

Fig. 6.2 Comparative characteristics of the spontaneous pre-ovulatory surges of FSH and LH [2]

6.2.2 The Stimulated Cycle

During ovarian stimulation procedures, a normal spontaneous gonadotropin surge of sufficient magnitude may result from the effect of rising estradiol levels in the presence of a mature dominant follicle that is primed to ovulate. This surge event usually occurs during a proper stimulation using pulsatile administration of GnRH or with oral clomiphene citrate, but gonadotropin treatment alone can also trigger a normal ovulation. The only drawback to this event is that it disorganizes plans for an in utero insemination, since the precise moment of the initiating gonadotropin rise becomes uncertain.

On the other hand, a triggered ovulation may not occur spontaneously during a cycle stimulated with gonadotropins, even in the presence of a mature follicle. For one thing the hypothalamic-pituitary-gonadal axis may be disrupted by supra-physiologic levels of estradiol. In addition, erratic gonadotropin surges of low magnitude and duration that are still incapable of initiating the complete ovulatory process may induce a premature luteinization of the follicle and/or a secretory transformation of the endometrium. Either event will adversely affect chances for a successful pregnancy. For these important reasons an ovulation should be medically triggered as soon as the follicular maturity criteria have been met.

6.3 Therapeutic Triggering of Ovulation

The triggering of ovulation is a crucial moment of the treatment. If done too early, the selected follicle may be still immature, and follicular rupture may not occur, or it may be difficult to fertilize the oocyte. If done too late, the follicle may be hypermature, leading to the same consequences. Judging follicular maturity criteria requires both morphological and functional assessment.

6.3.1 Sonographic Criteria

6.3.1.1 Follicular Diameter

The mean diameter of a mature follicle is typically between 16 and 23 mm. Although there are no clear-cut data in the literature, it is claimed that this optimal diameter can vary in accordance with the specific gonadotropin preparation used for the stimulation: a bit larger with HMG use (average 18 mm) than with FSH use (average 16 mm), and both being lesser than when clomiphene is used (average >20 mm) [7]. However, one study has shown that the pregnancy rate when using HMG was comparable when the mean dominant follicular diameter was only 16 mm or larger at the time of hCG administration [8].

6.3.1.2 Uterine Mucosa

The endometrium itself must be anechogenic, in three distinct leaves, and with the "coffee bean" appearance. Thickness should optimally reach at least 7 mm, although a successful nidation may occasional settle on a slightly thinner mucosa.

6.3.1.3 Hormonal Criteria

The level of secreted estradiol, by the dominant follicle(s) as well as the smaller ones, depends on the stimulation protocol. Expect levels to be greater than those in the normal physiologic pre-ovulatory phase:

- For a monofollicular stimulation, estradiol should be between 150 and 350 pg/ ml.
- For a paucifollicular stimulation, estradiol levels will be much higher, between 500 and 800–1,000 pg/ml, and are dependent on the number of dominant follicles.
- For multifollicular stimulations (or COH), estradiol level is also a function of the number of follicles to be punctured, and should run between 70 and 140 pg/ml per follicle >14 mm diameter [9]. The only remaining matter of debate concerns these upper values that seem to vary among different clinicians in accordance with their own perception of the risks of hyperstimulation. The upper limit of safety is typically acknowledged to be 2,500 pg/ml, although some clinicians accept upper ranges in excess of 5,000 pg/ml.

6.3.2 Chorionic Gonadotropin

Pituitary LH has never been available in clinical practice for procedures of triggering ovulation. This role has been relegated to placental hCG since the earliest days of ovulation stimulation, when PMSG was the sole available FSH product. Chorionic gonadotropin is without effect on the resting ovary. It may provoke follicular atresia or luteinization when administered during the early part of the menstrual cycle, and of course it exerts a trophic effect on the corpus luteum when administered during the luteal phase. This latter action is able to extend the functional life of a corpus luteum unless it is has already begun to wane. When administered in the presence of a mature follicle, hCG triggers ovulation no matter the gonadotropin that had been used to stimulate development. It is quite paradoxical that, despite considerable progress in strategies for ovulatory stimulation that closely mimic the physiologic process, the use of "nonphysiologic" hCG to trigger the actual ovulation has never been questioned, either in principle or in practice. In fact, the main natural hormone for triggering physiologic ovulation is LH, in association with FSH, and LH indeed exhibits numerous distinctions from hCG.

6.3.3 LH and hCG

Both of these hormones are glycoprotein heterodimers sharing the same alpha subunit but having unique beta subunits, although the primary sequences of beta LH and hCG subunits are actually the most closely homologous (96 %) of all glycoprotein hormones. Both complete hormones also possess a high degree of specificity for the same receptor (LH-hCG-R). The sequence of the hCG-β subunit includes a chain of 31 additional amino acids at the carboxyl-terminal end, and increased sialic

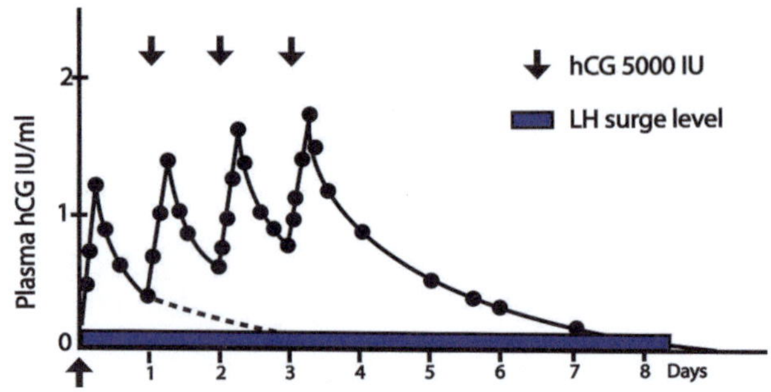

Fig. 6.3 Plasma accumulation of hCG following repeated administration [13]

acid content also contributes to a greater molecular mass. Because of this hCG has a slower hepatorenal degradation, a slower renal elimination rate and thus a longer plasma half-life. A partial desyalization of hCG brings its pharmacodynamic properties as well as its clinical effects in closer alignment to those of LH [10].

The elimination curve of both hormones is bi-exponential. LH shows an initial rapidly decreasing phase of about 45 min half-life (versus 8 h for hCG), followed by a second slower decline of some 10 h (versus 35–56 h for hCG). Recombinant hormone and extracted preparations have the same elimination curves as natural hormone [11]. The slow elimination of hCG explains why the hormone is still detectible for as long as 2 weeks following a 10,000 IU administration, and this property assuredly complicates interpretation of a standard pregnancy test one might conduct following a triggered ovulation [12]. In addition, the slower elimination rate assures that a single administration of hCG will be capable of providing a comparable or longer LH-like action to an endogenous pre-ovulatory gonadotropin surge. Repeated daily injections of hCG will cause a progressive accumulation in plasma, especially when administered by the IM route. Thus repeated hCG administration runs a risk for a hyperstimulation syndrome, without enhancing the clinical efficacy (Fig. 6.3) [13].

Commercially extracted urinary hCG is very heterogeneous: preparations may contain as much as 45 % chain fragments having little or no activity, with significant batch-to-batch variations [14]. On the other hand, the development of a recombinant hCG has ended with a product consisting of 100 % complete hormone.

6.3.4 Triggering Ovulation with hCG

In the past, programs of ovarian stimulation with gonadotropins would trigger ovulation with one to several hCG doses of 1,000–3,000 IU each, administered either simultaneously with or shortly following the final HMG injection. The only true advance in this design came in the early 1960s when hCG administration was reduced to one single dose, usually on the day *after* the last FSH injection.

The basic issue regarding the precise dose that is both necessary and sufficient to trigger an adequate ovulation has really never been resolved, undoubtedly because of the absence of recognizable side effects when unnecessarily high hCG doses are used. Nevertheless it has been documented with animal studies that excessive hCG dosing can induce a rather brutal luteinization of the dominant follicle, leading to a LUF syndrome [15]. Brown described an hCG threshold, similar to that for FSH, and did not hesitate to give 40,000–60,000 IU hCG for triggering ovulation in some patients, although this was done prior to the availability of ultrasound monitoring [16]. Nevertheless it would seem useful to address the question of an optimal dose, at least on the theoretical level.

Basic principles of endocrinology practice hold an exact quantity of any administered hormone should be determined in order to produce a precise effect. In other words, what is true for FSH administration should be the same for hCG. It seems archaic to decide that an appropriate dose of hCG to trigger ovulation relies on little more than the patient characteristics and the stimulation intensity.

However, more out of habit than from solid scientific evidence, the typical hCG dosing level has become:

- Approximately 5,000 IU for a mono- or paucifollicular stimulation
- Approximately 5,000–10,000 IU in COH

Work published by Abdallah indicated that although a dose of 10,000 IU does not provide a significant benefit in comparison to 5,000 IU in COH protocols, the lower doses may still be insufficient in some patients [17]. The bioavailable level of hCG is a function of the injected dose but also of the patient's BMI. A 5,000 IU dose may result in fewer harvested oocytes and diminish the chances for a successful pregnancy in the obese patient [18].

It is nevertheless well established that the different steps of the ovulatory process do require different amounts of hCG for optimal completion. Whereas lesser amounts should be sufficient to resume meiosis and an adequate oocyte maturity, higher doses are required for actual follicular rupture, and still higher levels are needed to establish and maintain a fully functional corpus luteum [19]. This is the reason why stimulation models used for IVF, where follicular puncture for ovum retrieval replaces the hormone-induced rupture, and where the luteal phase is supported by exogenous progesterone administration, have turned out to be inadequate for ovulation triggering in classic stimulation protocols, where lower doses may be sufficient. We have demonstrated that doses of 5,000, 3,000 or even 1,500 IU uhCG can provide comparable results regarding frequency of the follicular rupture, plasma progesterone levels, length of the luteal phase and pregnancy success rates [20]. Indeed, an adequate ovulatory process may even be triggered with 500 IU hCG administered intravenously [21]. In the practical sense, a 5,000 IU dose of extracted hCG seems sufficient for triggering ovulation following a classical (non-COH) stimulation with gonadotropins, and for guarding against possible variations of batch-to-batch bioactivity.

There has been considerable hope that the synthesis of rhCG (choriogonadotropin alpha, Ovidrel®) would finally provide an opportunity for precise characterization of appropriate doses for each type of stimulation protocol, and to modify some old habits long unsupported by scientific validation. Unfortunately this has not occurred, offering more evidence of the complete lack of interest on the part of the clinical-scientific community in menstrual cycle events occurring after the administration of hCG. The strategy of determining appropriate rhCG doses has merely attempted to approximate the plasma elimination curve of uhCG, and has resulted in release of only one dosage size at 250 μg, equivalent to 5,000–6,500 IU uhCG. This has at least pleased both supporters of the 5,000 and 10,000 IU doses. On the other hand, administration of a double-sized dose of rhCG (i.e., 500 μg) significantly enhances the risk for OHSS without bringing a superior clinical outcome [22].

6.3.5 hCG Administration and Follicular Rupture

Complete follicular rupture, as documented by ultrasound, actually takes place over a lengthy period of time following a single I.M. administration of hCG. With a mean time interval of about 40 h, follicular rupture occurs prior to the 36th hour in only 10 % of cycles, and not until after 48 h in another 10 % of cycles [21]. These time intervals following hCG administration are comparable to those observed from the beginning of the endogenous pre-ovulatory surge of gonadotropins, characterized by an LH surge initiating rise (LH-SIR) [3].

In clinical practice, however, the precise knowledge of the very moment of the follicular rupture is paradoxically of little help to assure success of the treatment cycle: other poorly understood parameters seem to be involved in the pregnancy rate, such as the penetration and survival of the spermatozoa within the cervical mucus, the duration of the spermatozoa fertilizing ability in vivo, and of the oocyte fecundability. For example, a large retrospective study reported comparable pregnancy rates if intra-uterine insemination occurred between the 28th and the 48th hours post-hCG (or within that same duration from the beginning of a spontaneous gonadotropin surge). Results were significantly lower for less than 28 h [23]. On the other hand, the pregnancy rate seems higher when performing insemination during the first day rather than the second after the LH rise [24]. Optimal intervals were even less well defined for the intra-cervical insemination, where the behavior of the spermatozoa within the cervical mucus becomes an important factor. Pregnancy rate was comparable when the insemination occurred on the same day or following day after of the hCG administration. Of course, a single programmed intercourse should occur within the same time interval.

6.3.6 Luteinizing Hormone

Using LH itself for triggering ovulation would avoid a number of potential hazards of hCG administration. This could be achieved either by mobilizing the pituitary gonadotroph LH pool, found in essentially all stimulated patients, with gonadorelin (GnRH) or a GnRH agonist (GnRHa), or by administration of recombinant LH itself.

6.3.6.1 Endogenous LH

Administration of hypothalamic GnRH mobilizes an initial burst of stored FSH and LH, and a gonadotropin surge that is capable of triggering ovulation of a mature follicle; this strategy has been studied since GnRH agonists first became available. However, this kind of induced surge is capable of inducing a significant proportion of abnormal luteal phases.

Regardless of the particular short-lived agonist used, a single administration results in a gonadotropin surge with a characteristic profile. Initially, a synchronous peak for both FSH and LH is reached within 4 h, at median levels of 150 and 45 IU/l for LH and FSH, respectively. From that point levels decrease gradually and return to baseline within 24 h in most patients (Fig. 6.4). This profile is quite different from the normal endogenous pre-ovulatory gonadotropin surge in that it begins more quickly, rises to higher peaks, and terminates sooner (Fig. 6.5). Nevertheless, a single administration of a short-lived GnRH agonist provides the same chance for a successful pregnancy as an injection of hCG, whether in a classical or a COH stimulation protocol [25].

Triggering with a GnRHa is relatively uncomplicated because a maximum gonadotropin surge will likely be elicited with a very modest dose. One vial of triptorelin (Decapeptyl®, 0.1 mg) administered sc, a single nasal spray of nafarelin (Synarel®, 0.2 mg), a single spray (0.1 mg) or sc injection (0.3 mg) of buserelin (Suprefact®), or a 0.2 mg sc dose of leuprolide (Lucrin®) are equally effective [26]. Higher doses than these do not result in a higher gonadotropin surge because the pituitary response is already maximized (Fig. 6.6).

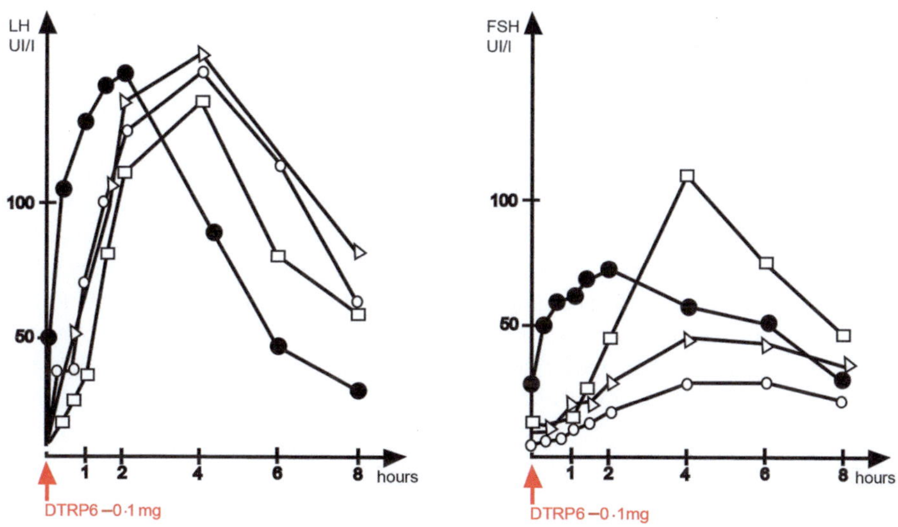

Fig. 6.4 FSH and LH surges elicited by a GnRH short-acting agonist in four patients (DTRP 60.1 = Triptorelin, 0.1 mg)

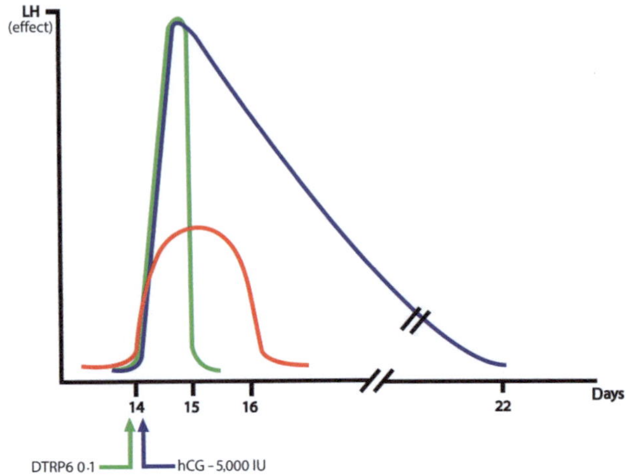

Fig. 6.5 LH effect following administration of a short-acting GnRH agonist or of hCG, contrasted with an endogenous pre-ovulatory gonadotropin surge (*in red*)

The principal benefit of triggering ovulation using GnRH is the significant reduction of risk for early ovarian hyperstimulation, due to the relatively shorter duration of LH effect upon the stimulated ovary. Some authors have reported no reluctance to trigger ovulation in IVF cycles when plasma estradiol was in excess of 15,000 pg/ml, and with no instances of early OHSS being observed [27]. The risk for multiple pregnancies also appears to be significantly decreased for the same reason: the gonadotropin surge triggers ovulation exclusively on a follicle of optimal maturity, whereas the prolonged duration of administered hCG action enables a greater number of dominant follicles to arrive at this critical maturity level and then to ovulate.

However, although the literature contains many reports as just described, it must be kept in mind that total elimination of the hyperstimulation hazard has not been completely validated through prospective studies, evidently for reasons of feasibility. Another point of caution is that while triggering with GnRH seems to avoid early hyperstimulation, this approach has only a minimal ability to prevent a late hyperstimulation following the appearance of hCG from an implanting embryo. Furthermore, the main drawback of triggering ovulation with a GnRH agonist is the tendency to produce a shortened or inadequate luteal phase in about one-third of the cycles, at least in some patients [28]. This insufficiency may be secondary to the shorter duration of the induced gonadotropin surge in comparison with the normal physiologic pre-ovulatory peak, or it may be caused by a temporary refractoriness of pituitary gonadotrophs and/or the luteal gland. Use of micronized oral progesterone seems to offers little improvement in these cases, and correction of this disorder is best accomplished through the administration of a low dose (750 to 1500 IU) of hCG. This, however, returns the risk of hyperstimulation.

6.3.6.2 Recombinant LH

The ability to trigger ovulation with exogenous pituitary LH following HMG stimulation has been established since 1964. However, extracted, purified human

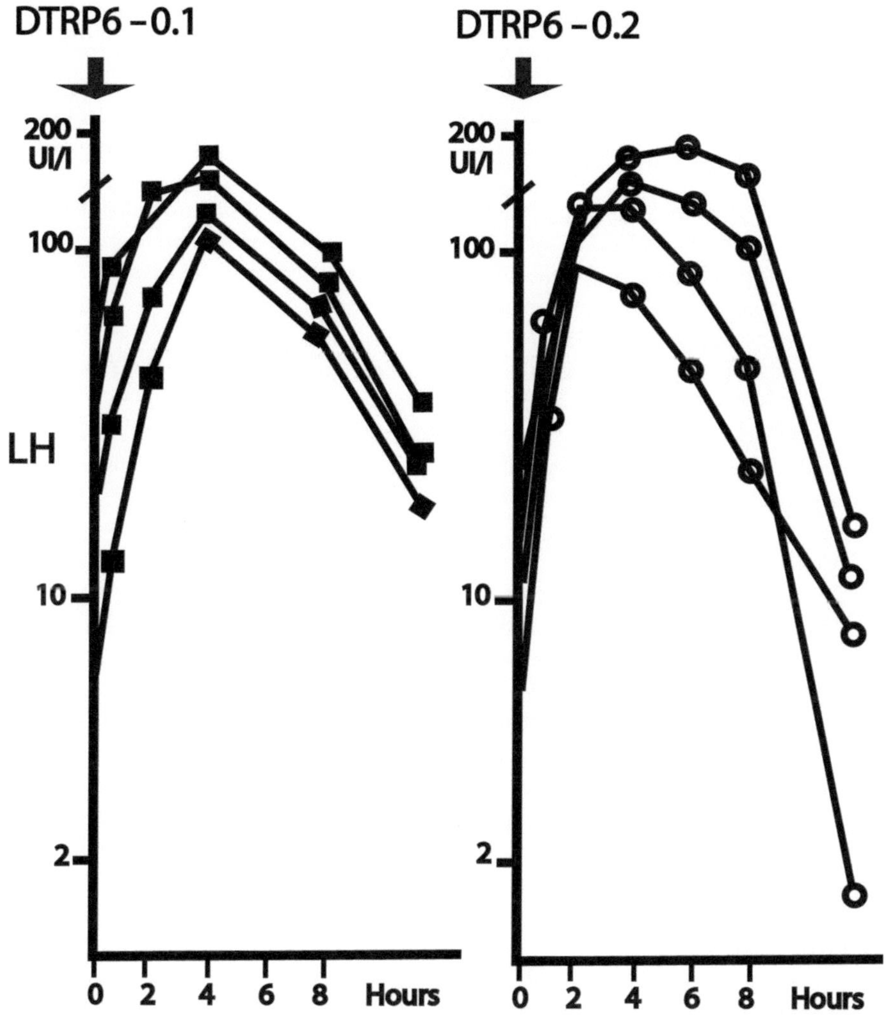

Fig. 6.6 Gonadotropin surges elicited by two different doses of a short-acting GnRH agonist (DTRP6 = Triptorelin). The responses were not greater when the dose was doubled, from 0.1 to 0.2 mg

pituitary hormone has never been made available for clinical use, and the question of LH administration in the clinic has appeared only in recent years following the announced synthesis of recombinant LH. This synthetic hormone has identical pharmacokinetic properties as extracted urinary and human pituitary LH. However, the issue of appropriate dosage has yet to be resolved. It has been established for LH, as it has for hCG, that progressively increasing quantities are needed to stimulate in turn the resumption of meiosis, follicular rupture, and then its transformation into a corpus luteum.

It appears that any single dose between 15,000 and 30,000 IU rLH will be sufficient to resume meiosis in a COH protocol [29]. In a classical stimulation, however, where LH must support the complete ovulatory process, results from studies in nonhuman primates suggested that a second administration of 2,500 IU 18 h after the first was necessary to complete an LH effect over the 48–50 h required to rupture a follicle and develop a functional luteal gland [30]. Obviously, these results suggest that inadequate LH exposure may lead to a luteal insufficiency or a LUF syndrome. In contrast, an excessive or a prolonged LH exposure creates the potential for the same risks as an hCG overdose. In one notable case, a quintuple pregnancy occurred after repeated high dosing with pituitary LH over 5 days [31].

It should also be mentioned that the practical question of using rLH to trigger ovulation is essentially moot because of high cost. Thus it seems highly unlikely that rLH, the only physiological product capable of reducing the risks for ovarian hyperstimulation as well as multiple pregnancy will ever be commercially available for triggering ovulation.

6.3.6.3 Oxytocin

This posterior pituitary hormone has a vast range of physiological effects outside its well-known actions to promote labor and milk ejection; among them is a possible role in fertility, particularly in the ovulatory process. Oxytocin receptors are present in cumulus and luteal cells of the ovary, and a 7-fold rise of plasma oxytocin occurs simultaneously with the pre-ovulatory LH surge. Administration of 5 IU oxytocin in the presence of a mature follicle in anovulatory women yields the same pregnancy rates as 5,000 IU hCG, apparently by triggering an endogenous LH surge [32]. This recent report was only a feasibility study, and the true value of this triggering mode, as well as its ability to prevent OHHS, particularly important in COH protocols, remains to be determined.

Conclusion

The process of triggering of ovulation is most assuredly as important as that of stimulating follicular growth, and it definitely requires as much care. Both a post-ovulatory measure of plasma progesterone and an ultrasound procedure to verify follicular rupture are recommended in order to reveal any hidden ovulatory dysfunctions that might help explain repeated failure to conceive following apparently successful ovarian stimulation cycles. To this point, nearly all of the research and developmental advances in ovulation induction have concerned exclusively the follicular stimulation, and the ovulation triggering step using hCG remains as an archaic reminder of an earlier era. Unfortunately, an endogenous LH surge cannot occur in every stimulation protocol, and recombinant LH will not likely ever be available for this indication. Thus the road remains open for continued use of hCG, either as an extracted or a recombinant product, along with its untoward trail of hazards and misfortune [33, 34].

References

1. Franchimont F, Hazee-Hagelstein MT, Charlet-Renard B et al (1994) Some basic mechanisms of ovulation. In: Emperaire JC (ed) The triggering of ovulation in stimulated cycles: HCG or LH? The Parthenon Publishing Group, London, pp 13–20
2. Hoff JD, Quidgley ME, Yen SSC (1983) Hormonal dynamics at mid-cycle: a reevaluation. J Clin Endocrinol Metab 57:792–796
3. Testard J, Frydman R, Feinstein MC et al (1998) Interpretation of plasma luteinizing hormone assay for the collection of mature oocytes from women: definition of a luteinizing hormone surge initiating rise. Fertil Steril 36:50–54
4. Cohlen BJ, TeVelde ER, Scheffer G et al (1993) The pattern of the luteinizing hormone surge in spontaneous cycles is correlated to the probability of conception. Fertil Steril 60:413–417
5. Bianchi V, Dal Prato L, Maccolini A et al (2009) Inadvertent recombinant follicle stimulating hormone bolus instead of human chorionic gonadotropin leads to the retrieval of competent oocytes in IVF program. Fertil Steril 92:1747.e1–1747.e3
6. Lamb JD, Shen S, McCulloch C et al (2011) Follicle stimulating hormone administered at the time of human chorionic gonadotropin trigger improves oocyte developmental competence in in vitro fertilization cycles: a randomized, double-blind, placebo-controlled trial. Fertil Steril 95:1655–1660
7. Shalom-Paz E, Marzal A, Wiser A et al (2014) Does optimal follicular size vary between clomiphene citrate and gonadotropin treatments? Gynecol Endocrinol 30:107–110
8. Da Silva A, Arbo E, Franchin R (2012) Early versus late HMG administration in mild-stimulated IUI cycles: a randomized clinical trial. Eur J Obstet Gynecol Reprod Biol 164:156–160
9. Loumaye E, Engrand P, Howles CM, O'Dean L (1997) An assessment of the role of serum luteinizing hormone and estradiol response to follicle stimulating hormone on the in vitro fertilization treatment outcome. Fertil Steril 67:889–899
10. Crosignani PG, Donini P (1994) The triggering of ovulation with partially desialylated HCG in HMG-stimulated cycles. In: Emperaire JC (ed) The triggering of ovulation in stimulated cycles: hCG or LH? The Parthenon Publishing Group, New York, pp 99–102
11. Le Cotonnec JY, Porchet HC, Beltrami V, Munafo A (1998) Clinical pharmacology of human luteinizing hormone. Part I. Pharmacokinetics after intravenous administration to healthy female volunteers and comparison with urinary human luteinizing hormone. Fertil Steril 69:189–194
12. Damewood MD, Shen W, Zacur HA et al (1989) Disappearance of exogenously administered human chorionic gonadotropin. Fertil Steril 52:398–402
13. Rizkallah T, Gurpide E, Van De Wiele RL (1969) Metabolism of HCG in man. J Clin Endocrinol Metab 29:92–100
14. Morse JH, Lustbader JW, Harrington JW, Canfield RE (1988) Heterogeneity of proteins in commercial preparations of human chorionic gonadotropin (hCG) demonstrated by western blotting. Am J Reprod Immunol 17:134–140
15. Bomsel-Helmreich O, Vun Nuyen L, Durand-Gasselin I (1989) Effects of varying doses of HCG on the evolution of preovulatory rabbit follicles and oocytes. Hum Reprod 4:636–642
16. Brown JB (1978) Pituitary control of ovarian function – concepts derived from gonadotrophin therapy. Aust N Z J Obstet Gynaecol 18:47–54
17. Abdallah H, Ah-Moye M (1987) The effect of the dose of HCG and the type of gonadotropin stimulation on oocyte recovery rate. Fertil Steril 48:958–963
18. Salha O, Dada T, Sharma V (2001) Influence of body mass index and self-administration of HCG on the outcome of IVF cycles: a prospective cohort study. Hum Fertil 4:37–42
19. Zelinski-Wooten MB, Hutchison JS, Trinchard-Lugan I et al (1997) Initiation of periovulatory events in gonadotropin-stimulated macaques with various doses of recombinant human chorionic gonadotropin. Hum Reprod 12:1877–1885

20. Emperaire JC, Parneix I, Broussin B, Ruffie A (1998) Triggering ovulation with different doses of human chorionic gonadotropin (hCG) in stimulated cycles. In: 16th World Congress on Fertility and Sterility, San Francisco, Abstr O-147, p 55
21. Fischer RA, Nakajima ST, Gibson M, Brumsted JR (1993) Ovulation after intravenous and intramuscular human chorionic gonadotropin. Fertil Steril 60:413–417
22. Chan CC, Ng EH, Tang OS et al (2005) A prospective, randomized double-blind study to compare two doses of recombinant human chorionic gonadotropin in inducing final oocyte maturity and the hormonal profile during the luteal phase. J Clin Endocrinol Metab 90:3933–3938
23. Fuh KW, Wang X, Tai A et al (1997) Intra-uterine insemination: effect of temporal relationship between the luteinizing hormone surge, human chorionic gonadotropin administration, and insemination on pregnancy rates. Hum Reprod 12:2162–2166
24. Blockeel C, Knez J, Polyzos NP et al (2014) Should an intra-uterine insemination with donor semen be performed 1 or 2 days after the spontaneous LH rise? A prospective RCT. Hum Reprod 29:697–703
25. Emperaire JC (1994) Le declenchement therapeutique de l'ovulation: vers le remplacement de l'HCG par la LH. Contracept Fertil Sexual 22:459–467
26. Parneix I, Emperaire JC, Ruffie A (2001) Comparaison de differents protocoles de declenchement ovulatoire par les agonistes de la GnRH et la gonadotrophine chorionique. Gynecol Obstet Fertil 29:100–115
27. Iliodromiti S, Lan VT, Tuong HM et al (2013) Impact of GnRH agonist triggering and extensive luteal support on live-birth rates and ovarian hyperstimulation syndrome: a retrospective cohort study. J Ovarian Res 6:93
28. Emperaire JC, Parneix I, Ruffie A (2004) Luteal phase defects following agonist-triggered ovulation: a patient-dependent response. Reprod Biomed Online 9:22–27
29. The European Recombinant LH Study Group (2001) The recombinant luteinizing hormone is as effective as, but safer than, urinary human chorionic gonadotropin in inducing final follicular maturation and ovulation in in vitro fertilization procedures: results of a multicenter double-blind study. J Clin Endocrinol Metab 86:2607–2618
30. Chandrasekher YA, Hutchison JS, Zelinski-Wooten MB et al (1994) Initiation of periovulatory events in primate follicles using recombinant and native human luteinizing hormone to mimic the mid-cycle gonadotropin surge. J Clin Endocrinol Metab 79:298–306
31. Jewelewicz R, James SL, Finster M et al (1972) Quintuplet gestation after ovulation induction with menopausal gonadotropins and pituitary luteinizing hormone. Obstet Gynecol 40:1–5
32. Mehrotra S, Singh U, Gupta HP et al (2014) A prospective double blind study comparing the effects of oxytocin and human chorionic gonadotrophin as trigger for ovulation. J Obstet Gynecol 34:13–16
33. Emperaire JC, Edwards RG (2004) Time to revolutionize the triggering of ovulation. Reprod Biomed Online 9:480–483
34. Emperaire JC (2005) Pourquoi continuer à tolérer l'hyperstimulation ovarienne? Gynecol Obstet Fertil 33:281–282
35. Caraty A, Evans NP, Fabre-Nys CJ, Karsch EJ (1995) The periovulatory gonadotropin-releasing hormone surge: a neuroendocrine signal for ovulation. J Reprod Fertil Suppl 49:245–255

Supporting the Luteal Phase

7

The luteal phase extends from the moment of ovulation triggering until the beginning of menses, or of pregnancy. The corpus luteum is generated from luteinized granulosa and theca interna cells that remained in the follicle after oocyte extrusion. It secretes both estrogens and progesterone under the effect of a pulsatile LH stimulation that is slower (3–5 pulses/24 h) than during the follicular phase (one pulse every 90 min). If conception and nidation follow ovulation, hCG secreted by the embryonic pouch maintains the luteal gland trophicity for secretion of both steroid classes (Fig. 7.1). Between the fifth and the seventh weeks of pregnancy the placenta also begins to assume autonomous synthesis and secretion of these hormones. Csapo showed in 1973 that the pregnancy was interrupted if the corpus luteum was removed earlier than the seventh week, but progesterone administration could rescue the pregnancy by this time [1].

In a natural menstrual cycle, a corpus luteum will typically produce 25–50 mg of progesterone daily, to maintain plasma levels at a mid-phase range of 10–20 ng/ml [2, 3]. Luteal phase defects may compromise the chances for pregnancy during the cycle leading to fertilization. Whereas there is little consensus regarding precise definitions (examples: short luteal phase of <10 days, plasma progesterone of <10 ng/ml, discrepancies between chronologic and endometrial dating in relation to the LH surge or to the previous menses), defects of the luteal phase are believed to be responsible for infertility in some 8 % of normally cycling patients. This type of dysfunction may be obviated by progesterone administration to induce a secretory transformation of the endometrium, thereby enhancing uterine mucosa receptivity to implantation, and by inhibiting uterine contractions [4].

Luteal phase defects are often secondary to an abnormal follicular development during the first part of the cycle, or to an inadequate pre-ovulatory surge of gonadotropins. This may explain how the process of directed ovarian stimulation can become involved in the quality of the resulting corpus luteum, and it also raises the question of efficacy of luteal supplementation. Luteal gland abnormalities appear to vary according to the type of ovarian stimulation. Whereas luteal insufficiencies are often documented following a COH with GnRH analogues, their appearance

J.-C. Emperaire, *Ovulation Stimulation with Gonadotropins*,
DOI 10.1007/978-3-319-18654-2_7

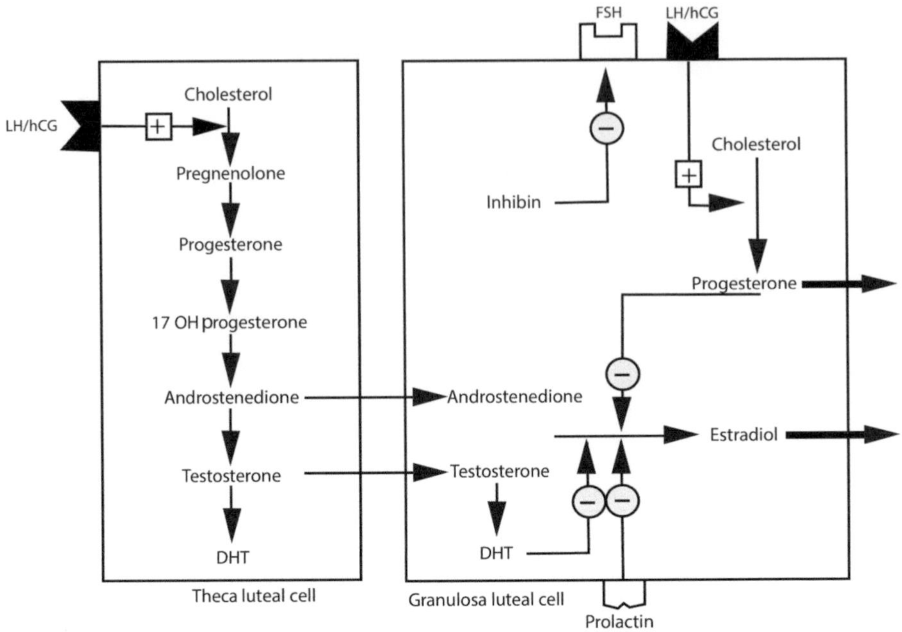

Fig. 7.1 Steroidogenesis in the corpus luteum, illustrating the contributions of separate compartments of theca and granulosa cells

following other stimulation conditions remains controversial and relies more on beliefs, habits, or some contradictory uncontrolled studies. The whole issue of maintaining luteal function also remains important on numerous fronts, as evidenced by a recent report that appears to link the occurrence of certain cancers in childhood with the administration of progesterone to the mother [5].

7.1 Luteal Phase Defects Following a Classic (Mono-to Paucifollicular) Stimulation

There are two types of scenario, depending upon the presence or the absence of an endogenous pulsatile LH secretion.

7.1.1 Normal Gonadotropins in Ovulation and Anovulation

An inadequate luteal phase can develop in a patient having a normal hypothalamic-pituitary-ovarian axis in two basic ways:

- A suboptimal follicular stimulation process leading to a granulosa cell population that remains insufficient for transformation to an adequate luteal gland. In this case, the luteal insufficiency could have been prevented with a more robust follicular stimulation.

- When hCG is used to trigger ovulation, there can be a temporary depression of LH pulsatility and secretion due to a short loop feedback. This has been identified under experimental conditions following hCG administration, and it can deprive the corpus luteum of sufficient LH stimulation [6]. However, this scenario has not been definitively identified in normally ovulating women [7]. Moreover, the action of a single hCG injection on the luteal gland typically persists for several days and should compensate for any temporary shortfall of LH secretion.

In fact, the standard practice of progesterone administration following a simple ovarian stimulation is not supported by study data. Reports are unable to establish its validity even after COH without analogues [8]. Luteal support also seems unnecessary following a single antagonist administration for insemination purposes [9]. On the other hand, progesterone administration may be mandatory in certain other situations, such as treating a short luteal phase (<10 days) or a when a post-ovulatory progesterone level remains under 10 ng/ml.

Two other points that are worthy of attention:

- Progesterone administration should not be started within 2 days of an hCG injection so that the integrity of the thinner pre-ovulatory cervical mucus will not be disturbed.
- Triggering ovulation with a GnRH agonist instead of hCG produces a short or inadequate luteal phase in about a third of the cycles, in certain patients. In those instances luteal support with progesterone is mandatory, or even better when combined with a single low dose of hCG (750 IU) 2–3 days after ovulation [10].

7.1.2 Hypogonadotropic Anovulation

In cases of primary or secondary pituitary insufficiency, supporting corpus luteum steroidogenesis becomes mandatory because LH secretion is definitely inadequate or possibly absent. When stimulation is conducted with a GnRH pump, the pulsatile gonadorelin administration should be continued for 7–10 days following ovulation. When stimulation is conducted with a gonadotropin preparation containing FSH and LH, luteal support should be provided either as progesterone or by injections of 1,500 IU hCG given three times at 3-day intervals [11]. In our experience, absence of luteal support does not reduce the pregnancy rate, probably because of LH-like properties of the hCG used for triggering ovulation that remain active until the time for implantation.

7.2 Multifollicular (COH) Stimulation

Typically, luteal support with progesterone or hCG has been prescribed following COH since the early days of IVF, in order to increase the pregnancy rate by preventing a possible luteal insufficiency. This situation often occurs when large numbers of granulosa cells become aspirated together with the oocyte, and/or when supra-physiologic levels of secreted estrogens have suppressed LH secretion. Nevertheless it was extensively documented that additional luteal support was not necessary in stimulation protocols using clomiphene + HMG or HMG alone. The activity of a typical 10,000 IU hCG triggering dose on the corpora lutea usually persists through the implantation period [12].

This situation changed dramatically with the arrival of GnRH agonists, because their use in COH protocols was usually followed by luteal phase perturbations that decreased pregnancy rates [13]. This premature luteolysis is due mainly to the prolonged suppression of pulsatile LH secretion that is necessary to maintain corpus luteum activity and steroid hormone production. Administration of a long acting GnRH agonist can permanently suppress pituitary LH secretion, and even a short-acting agonist can suppress LH for 10–20 days following the final application.

7.2.1 Types of Luteal Support

Five substances are available for corpus luteum support, or as a substitute in case of its failure.

- *Chorionic gonadotropin*, which binds to the LH/hCG receptors of luteal cells and stimulates secretion of estradiol and progesterone. Continuing hCG administration during the post-ovulatory period provides a very effective support of luteal function, but it also carries a real risk for late ovarian hyperstimulation (OHSS). Repeated injections of hCG lead to an accumulation in plasma because of the hormone's prolonged prolonged half-life [14]. For this reason, this potentially hazardous yet effective method of support is not usually prescribed following COH with GnRH analogues. Progesterone administration provides the same quality of result without any risk for OHSS.

  On the other hand, when ovulation is triggered with a short acting GnRH agonist in an antagonist protocol, administration of a small dose of hCG (750–1,500 IU) is mandatory in order to regain a normal luteal phase and pregnancy rates; indeed, administration of progesterone alone or with estradiol, may not be sufficient [15].
- *Progesterone* administration is adequate for luteal support of COH stimulation cycles. Several routes of administration are possible, but each has certain drawbacks [16]:

  Vaginal suppositories of micronized progesterone are widely used at a 200–600 mg daily dose, but this may result in vaginal discharges with occasional local irritation.

  Vaginal 8 % progesterone gel (Crinone®), 90 mg daily, has the same efficacy and drawbacks as the suppositories.

  Intramuscular depot of 500 g progesterone in oil on the evening following oocyte retrieval, plus a second injection 7 days later, is effective. However, prolonged absorption of hormone from the injection site may result in menstrual cycle disorders for several months if a pregnancy is not achieved.

Intramuscular depot of smaller progesterone doses (*50 mg daily*) have much less potential for cycle disruption but this approach requires a series of daily administrations rather than a single large one.

Subcutaneous self-administration of aqueous progesterone (Prolutex®) has shown similar results to vaginal progesterone, but this product is not yet available in every country [17].

Oral dydrogesterone (Duphaston®) at a 20 mg daily dose provides a comfortable, effective luteal support, but is curiously seldom used [18].

None of the various progesterone preparations available in different countries appears to be superior to the others, and none is actually more efficacious than treatment with hCG [19].

- *Estradiol*: The exact role of the luteal secretion of estradiol remains hypothetical. During COH, estradiol reaches supra-physiologic levels that peak just before the hCG administration, then it rapidly decreases following oocyte retrieval and rises again during mid-luteal phase, much as in the normal menstrual cycle pattern. Following a report [20] that estradiol levels were higher 9–10 days after the ovulatory gonadotropin surge in conception cycles, interest appeared for supplementation with progesterone *and* estradiol during the luteal phase following COH. On the other hand, it remains debated whether a systematic 2–8 mg dose of oral micronized estradiol should be administered to patients whose endogenous estradiol levels have already exceeded the normal physiologic range [21]. Nevertheless, continued post-ovulatory monitoring of some patients will determine whether estradiol administration is advantageous. It has been proposed to use estradiol supplementation only in cycles where the plasma level falls below 100 pg/ml within 11 days after the embryo transfer [22].
- *GnRH agonists* are paradoxically able to improve the luteal phase in certain situations by provoking additional LH secretion. One approach is to continue with daily intranasal application of buserelin following a classic ovulation triggering with 200 μg of the same agonist. However, dosing must retreat below a level (e.g., 100 μg) that desensitizes the pituitary [23]. Another approach is to administer a single dose of 0.1 mg triptorelin 6 days after oocyte retrieval. This is reported to improve the implantation rate significantly, with effects on pituitary, the endometrium and possibly the embryo itself through their GnRH receptors [24]. This effect remains to be confirmed, and furthermore, one should be cautious when supporting the luteal phase with GnRH agonists following COH because effects of these peptides on the embryo are largely unknown. On the other hand, there are also reassuring reports of spontaneous conceptions during the activity period of long acting agonists [25].
- *Pituitary LH*: If a GnRH agonist is used to trigger ovulation during an antagonist COH protocol, progesterone alone will not be able to maintain the luteal phase. However, the addition of 300 IU recombinant LH (Luveris®) every other day is able to restore an adequate luteal phase. This would appear to confirm the belief that luteal abnormalities following COH with GnRH analogues result from an insufficient LH support [26]. Still, the cited report was only a feasibility study; the cost of recombinant hormone treatment in a clinical practice study would be excessively expensive in comparison with the administration of progesterone alone that would be expected to yield the same result [27].

7.2.2 When to Start?

Progesterone administration can be started on the day of triggering ovulation, on the day of oocyte retrieval (Day 0) or on the day of embryo transfer (Day 3) [28]. However, further delay does appear to diminish the pregnancy rate [29].

7.2.3 When to Stop?

Although various approaches coexist in this field, it is now fairly well understood that continuing luteal phase support beyond the first positive pregnancy test has essentially no effect upon the future course. The rates of chemical pregnancy, ectopic pregnancy, or spontaneous abortion are comparable whether progesterone administration is stopped on the first day of a positive pregnancy test, or continued on up through three more weeks, or even longer [30].

Conclusion

Luteal support is mandatory only following a COH with GnRH analogues. Whatever galenic formulation is chosen, progesterone is capable of restoring both luteal phase quality and normal pregnancy rates, except in the particular case of the agonist-triggered ovulation. Use of hCG is as effective as progesterone but this hormone increases the risk for secondary OHSS.

References

1. Csapo AL, Pulkinnen MO, Wiest WG (1973) Effects of luteectomy and progesterone replacement therapy in early pregnant patients. Am J Obstet Gynecol 115:759–765
2. Strauss JF, Williams CJ (2014) The ovarian life cycle. In: Strauss JF, Barbieri RL (eds) Yen & Jaffe's Reproductive Endocrinology, 7th edn. Elsevier Saunders, Philadelphia, pp 157–191
3. Sallam HN, Sallam A, Ezzeldin F et al (1999) Reference values for the midluteal plasma progesterone concentration: evidence from human menopausal gonadotropin- stimulated pregnancy cycles. Fertil Steril 71:711–714
4. Rosenberg SM, Luciano AA, Riddick DH (1980) The luteal phase defect: the relative frequency of, and encouraging response to, treatment with vaginal progesterone. Fertil Steril 34:17–20
5. Hargreave M, Jensen S, Nielsen TTS et al (2014) Maternal use of fertility drugs and risk for cancer in the childhood – a nationwide population based cohort study in Denmark. Int J Cancer 136(8):1931–1939
6. Miyake A, Aono T, Kinugasa T et al (1979) Suppression of serum levels of luteinizing hormone by short- and long-loop negative feedback in ovariectomized women. J Endocrinol 80:353–356
7. Tavianotou A, Devroey P (2003) Effect of human chorionic gonadotropin on luteal luteinizing hormone concentrations in natural cycles. Fertil Steril 80:654–655
8. Jones GS, Garcia A, Acosta A (1982) Luteal phase evaluation in *in vitro* fertilization. In: Edwards RG and Purdy JM (eds) Human Conception In Vitro, Academic Press, London, pp 297–310
9. Ragni G, Vegetti W, Baroni E et al (2001) Comparison of luteal phase profile in gonadotrophin stimulated cycles with or without a gonadotrophin-releasing hormone antagonist. Hum Reprod 16:2258–2262

10. Emperaire JC, Parneix I, Ruffie A (2004) Luteal phase defects following agonist-triggered ovulation: a patient-dependent response. Reprod Biomed Online 9:22–27
11. Dubourdieu S, Freour T, Dessolle L, Barriere P (2011) Prospective, randomized study of pulsatile GnRH therapy and gonadotropin treatment (FSH + LH) for ovulation induction in women with hypothalamic amenorrhea and underlying polycystic ovary syndrome. Fertil Steril 96(Suppl):S83
12. Daya S (1988) Efficacy of progesterone support in the luteal phase following *in vitro* fertilization and embryo transfer: meta-analysis of clinical trials. Hum Reprod 3:731–734
13. Smith J, Devroey P, Camus M et al (1988) The luteal phase and early pregnancy after combined GnRH agonist/HMG treatment for superovulation in IVF of GIFT. Hum Reprod 3:585–590
14. Rizkallah T, Gurpide E, Van De Wiele RL (1969) Metabolism of HCG in man. J Clin Endocrinol Metab 29:92–100
15. Humaidan P, Ejdrup Bredkjaer H, Westergaard LG, Yding Andersen C (2010) 1500 IU chorionic gonadotropin administered at oocyte retrieval rescues the luteal phase when gonadotropin-releasing hormone agonist is used for ovulation induction: a prospective randomized, controlled study. Fertil Steril 93:847–854
16. Hubayter ZR, Muasher SJ (2008) Luteal supplementation in *in vitro* fertilization: more questions than answers. Fertil Steril 89:749–758
17. Baker VL, Jones CA, Doody K et al (2014) A randomized, controlled trial comparing the efficacy and safety of aqueous subcutaneous progesterone with vaginal progesterone for luteal phase support in in vitro fertilization. Hum Reprod 10:2012–2020
18. Belaisch-Allart J, Testard J, Fries N et al (1987) The effect of dydrogesterone supplementation in an IVF program. Hum Reprod 2:183–185
19. Fatemi HM, Popvic-Todorovic B, Papanikolaou E et al (2007) An update of luteal phase support in stimulated IVF cycles. Hum Reprod Update 13:581–590
20. Zegers-Hochschild F, Altieri E (1995) Luteal estrogen is not required for the establishment of pregnancy in humans. J Assist Reprod Genet 12:224–228
21. Jee BC, Suh CS, Kim SH et al (2010) Effects of estradiol supplementation during the luteal phase of *in vitro* fertilization cycles: a meta-analysis. Fertil Steril 93:428–436
22. Kalder AS, Coulam CB (2000) Luteal estrogen supplementation in pregnancies associated with low serum estradiol concentrations. Early Pregnancy 4:191–199
23. Pirard C, Donnez J, Loumaye E (2005) GnRH agonist as novel luteal support: results of a randomized, parallel group feasibility study using intranasal administration of buserelin. Hum Reprod 20:1798–1804
24. Kyrou D, Kolibianakis EM, Fatemi HM et al (2011) Increased live birth rates with GnRH agonist addition for luteal support in ICSI/IVF cycles: a systematic review and meta-analysis. Hum Reprod Update 17:734–740
25. Lambalk CB, Homburg R (2006) GnRH agonist for luteal support in IVF? Setting the balance between enthusiasm and caution. Hum Reprod 21:2580–2582
26. Papanikolaou EG, Verpoest W, Fatemi H et al (2011) A novel method of luteal supplementation with recombinant luteinizing hormone when a gonadotropin-releasing hormone agonist is used instead of human chorionic gonadotropin for ovulation triggering: a randomized prospective proof of concept study. Fertil Steril 95:1174–1177
27. Kol S, Humaidan P, Itskovitz-Eldor J (2011) GnRH agonist ovulation trigger and HCG-based, progesterone-free luteal support: a proof of concept study. Hum Reprod 26:2874–2877
28. Mochtar MH, Van Wely M, Van Der Ven F (2006) Timing luteal phase support in GnRH agonist down-regulated IVF/embryo transfer cycles. Hum Reprod 21:905–908
29. Williams SC, Oehninger S, Gibbons WE et al (2001) Delaying the initiation of progesterone supplementation results in decreased pregnancy rates after *in vitro* fertilization: a randomized, prospective study. Fertil Steril 76:1140–1143
30. Proctor A, Hurst BS, Marshburn PB, Mathews ML (2006) Effect of progesterone supplementation in early pregnancy on the pregnancy outcome after *in vitro* fertilization. Fertil Steril 85:1550–1552

8 Avoiding Complications

Stimulating ovulation is a formidable procedure, and as such includes risk for complications commensurate with its intensity. One must always keep in mind the balance between expected benefits and predictable hazards. All aspects should be carefully explained to the couple who are, after all, the principal role players in this plan. Essentially all of the risk can be ascribed to excessive stimulation, of which there are two basic types: predictable problems, typically uncovered during a preliminary assessment of the couple's fertility parameters that may be considered as primary prevention, and unpredictable problems, which appear during the treatment (i.e., secondary prevention).

It is of course always possible to stop a stimulation cycle if and when conditions exceed the fixed limits. But deprogramming a cycle has a cost, at the least an emotional cost for the patient who has already committed to a number of injections, blood tests, and ultrasound examinations. Plus there is a financial cost that may vary according to the couple's health care plan. Thus both clinician and patient tend to be reluctant to drop out of a stimulation cycle and this is how consideration of hazard tends to become a notion of reasoned risk, or a presumed risk. Whereas some complications appear to be totally unexpected, even *a posteriori*, most are in fact objectively foreseeable. The weight of the human factor, which is clearly the most difficult factor to manage, remains of major importance.

8.1 Multiple Pregnancies

The risk for multiple pregnancies occurs only with classical mono- or paucifollicular stimulations. In controlled ovarian hyperstimulation for IVF purposes, multiple pregnancies result from transfer policies and not from the stimulation process itself.

J.-C. Emperaire, *Ovulation Stimulation with Gonadotropins*,
DOI 10.1007/978-3-319-18654-2_8

8.1.1 Monofollicular Stimulation

The purpose of monofollicular stimulation is to promote the development of only a single follicle, and then to trigger ovulation in the presence of a single mature follicle.

Effective primary prevention relies on the choice of the starting dose and the gonadotropin administration protocol:

8.1.1.1 Starting Dose

Even if the starting dose is incorrectly chosen, an insufficient dose remains easier to handle than an excessive dose. For this reason a lower dose (e.g., 50 IU) should be favored for starting a patient who has not previously received gonadotropins, especially when AMH levels and/or AFC are elevated. A higher dose (75 IU) may be considered for patients who are over 38 years of age or are overweight, yet it is not unreasonable to start with a lower dose even in those cases.

8.1.1.2 Administration Protocol

The classic "step up" protocol, with an initial assessment after 5 days of gonadotropin administration, is most suitable for ovulatory patients. In anovulatory patients, or in patients with elevated levels of AMH and/or AFC, lower dose increments are indicated after an initial trial of 7 days' treatment.

Effective secondary prevention includes adjusting the gonadotropin dosage and administration protocol in response to the patient's reactions, and with respect to appropriate triggering criteria. The initial protocol should be reconsidered after 5–7 days of administration, to be continued as a classic step-up, a step-up low dose, a chronic step-up low dose, or step-down protocol in some cases. Results of hormonal and ultrasound assessments adjust the gonadotropin doses and the number of administration days before the next assessment. The triggering criteria in monofollicular stimulation cycles are strict: a single follicle must be >15 mm diameter without other secondary follicle(s) >12 mm.

8.1.2 Bifollicular Stimulation

This strategy is used to elicit a second follicle and oocyte capable of being fertilized, to compensate for the patient's age, because of another hypofertility factor, or even in cases of an idiopathic infertility. This type of stimulation requires particular care, because a third (or even a fourth) follicle can be developed inadvertently.

Effective primary prevention in the spontaneously ovulating patient involves development of a second follicle either by recruiting a new one with an early stimulation (CD 3–5) at a low to mid-range dose (50–75 IU), or by rescuing a spontaneous secondary follicle with later stimulation (CD 6–7) at higher doses (75–1,125 IU). In anovulatory patients, the starting dose should be slightly higher than the posology that is sufficient for a single follicle, and the administration protocol should be careful to permit only two follicles to develop.

Secondary prevention relies on the triggering criteria, including the patient's age, the presence of secondary follicles, and the estradiol level, in order to balance the chances for conception against the risks for multiple pregnancy. A flow chart proposed by P. Barri appears to be an adequate decision strategy [1].

8.1.3 Paucifollicular Stimulation

Triggering ovulation in the presence of three or perhaps four mature follicles should be considered only in the patients over 40 years of age, whose chances for pregnancy, and also for multiple pregnancy, are significantly reduced.

8.2 Ovarian Hyper Stimulation Syndrome (OHSS)

OHSS is a potential complication for any stimulation cycle, classical as well as COH. Aside from a few situations such as a paradoxical effect of a GnRH agonist or in some cases of hyperthyroidism, OHSS appears exclusively due to hCG influence, no matter the timing of administration (Fig. 8.1). Early (or primary) OHSS tends to occur within the week following ovulation triggering. Late (or secondary) OHSS appears a few days before the next expected menses, due to the reappearance of endogenous hCG from an implanting embryo. Furthermore, a primary OHSS may be enhanced by a secondary hyperstimulation at the beginning of a pregnancy.

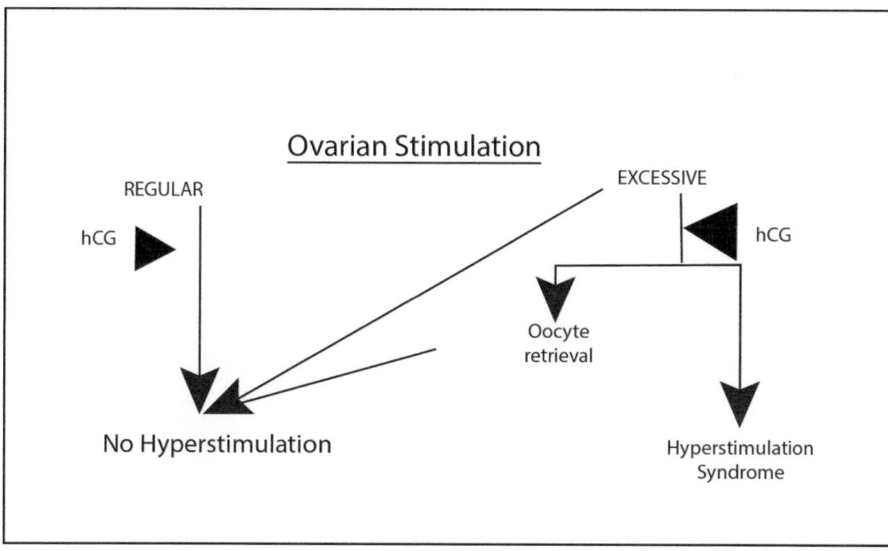

Fig. 8.1 Role of hCG in the genesis of the ovarian hyperstimulation syndrome: OHSS does not occur without hCG

8.2.1 Pathophysiology

OHSS is provoked by the secretion of vasoactive substances from granulosa cells under the influence of hCG. In particular, a vascular endothelial growth factor (VEGF-A) binds to the ovarian follicles and especially to vascular endothelial cells through two receptors (VGEF-R1 and 2). VEGF production increases throughout gonadotropin stimulation and reaches a peak within 48 h following the administration of hCG. These vasoactive substances induce angiogenesis, increase the permeability of capillary endothelium, and facilitate a net hydro-electrolytic shift from plasma to extravascular spaces (Fig. 8.2). These changes result in diminished intravascular volume and hemoconcentration, enhanced risk for hypercoagulation, hepatorenal failure, and can produce a massive fluid exudation with sequestration into extravascular spaces in the pelvic, abdominal, and even the pleural and pericardial cavities. The ovaries themselves increase in volume and develop functional cysts that can be hemorrhagic (Fig. 8.3). Occurrence of OHSS may also be facilitated by polymorphisms of VEGF and VEGF-R2 [2].

8.2.2 Grades of Ovarian Hyperstimulation

Three grades of OHSS are typically recognized, in accordance with clinical symptoms and the degree of fluid effusion (Table 8.1).

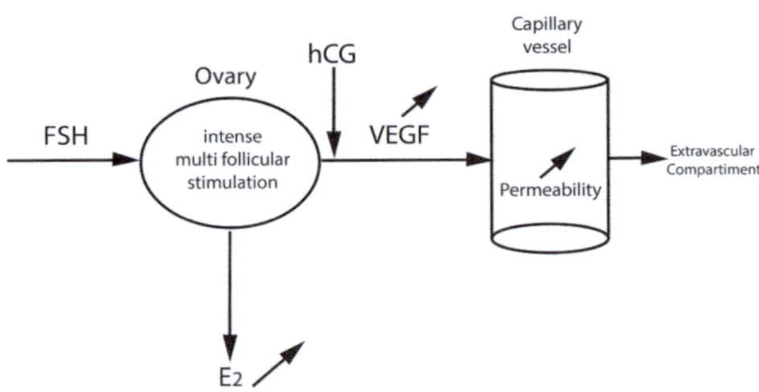

Fig. 8.2 Pathophysiology of OHSS: roles of hCG and VEGF

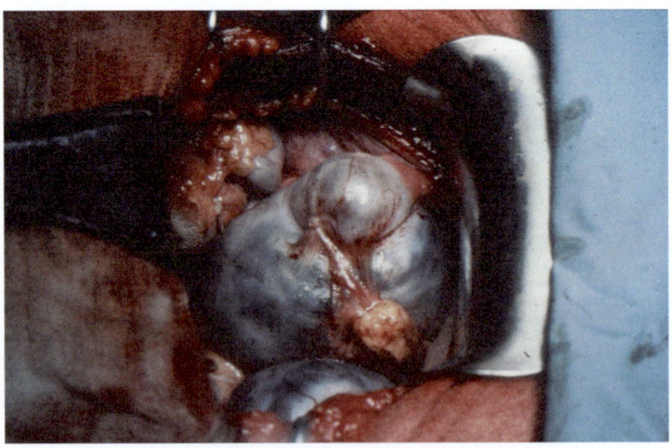

Fig. 8.3 Appearance at laparoscopy of hyperstimulated ovaries: note the hemorrhagic cysts (Photo courtesy RB Greenblatt)

Table 8.1 The three degrees of severity of OHSS [3, 4]

	OHSS		
	MILD	MODERATE	SEVERE
SUBJECTIVE CRITERIA			
Abdominal distension	+	+	+
Abdominal pain	+	+	+
Digestive disorders	±	±	±
Dyspnea			
Oliguria < 600 ml/day	−	±	+
OBJECTIVE CRITERIA			
ULTRASOUND Fluid Douglas pouch	+	+	+
Peri-utero-ovarian	−	+	+
Peri-intestinal	−	−	+
Pleural	−	−	+
ovarian volume (ml)	9-12	>12	>12
BIOLOGY			
Hematocrit %	< 45	45 -55	>55
White blood cells	< 15 000	15 000 -25 000	>25 000
Hypernatremia	−	−	+
Hypokaliemia	−	−	+
Creatinine > 1,5 mg/dL	−	−	±
Clotting disorders	−	−	±

Grade 1 (*mild*) is characterized by abdominal pain with digestive symptoms: nausea with or without vomiting and diarrhea, or possibly constipation. Ultrasonography reveals enlarged ovaries containing many cysts, in fact difficult to recognize from the picture usually seen following an oocyte harvest. Peritoneal effusion is also visible, limited to the Pouch of Douglas. Biologic parameters remain within the normal range.

Grade 2 (*moderate*) presents the same symptoms as Grade 1 with increased intensity and abdominal distension. Ultrasonography shows ovaries larger than 12 cm in the long axis, with ascites rising above the uterus. Common biologic alterations include a leukocytosis (WBC of 15–20,000) and a rise of hematocrit (but remaining <55 %). A possible torsion of the adnexa may be difficult to recognize in this situation.

Grade 3 (*severe*) encompasses increased ascites, and effusion that sometimes reaches the pleural cavity to create dyspnea. Oliguria can occur along with various abnormal lab findings, e.g., leukocytosis (>25,000), hemoconcentration (hematocrit >55 %), hyponatremia, hyperkalemia, and serum creatinine in the range of 1–1.5 mg/dl. The severity of the syndrome may lead to organ failures complicated with thrombotic events.

Mild and moderate OHSS typically recede spontaneously without after-effects, whereas severe OHSS may become life threatening and may require paracentesis. Intensive care hospitalization and anti-coagulation therapy currently provide effective management of these complications, yet it remains the case that the desire for a baby can still cost someone their life.

Although the development of OHSS is always related to the presence of hCG, the patient's overall condition can also be a contributing factor, making outcomes variable and uncertain. Even patients with very similar ultrasound and hormonal monitoring parameters prior to hCG administration may develop disparate degrees of OHSS afterwards. I have personally encountered a severe OHSS syndrome in the presence of a single mature follicle without evidence of secondary follicles and a with a plasma estradiol level of only 175 pg/ml. Furthermore, the prognosis of a beginning OHSS remains largely unknown. Plasma levels of total VEGF-A do not correlate strongly with the developing syndrome, but free VEGF-A does seem to be modestly reliable [5]. For all these reasons, it is always preferable to discontinue the cycle rather than to risk OHSS when the stimulation protocol exceeds proper limits.

8.2.3 Prevention of Ovarian Hyperstimulation Syndrome

Detection and management of OHSS operates on four levels [6]:

8.2.3.1 Primary Prevention

Aside from those patients who have been previously stimulated and whose susceptibility to gonadotropins is already known, detection of a potential risk for OHSS should include evaluation of her ovarian reserve along with three main criteria:

Age: Although ovarian sensitivity to gonadotropins decreases with age, an unexpectedly high response may occur in a patient over 38 years of age. For this reason, age should typically be considered as a secondary parameter when assessing risk.

Antral follicular count (*AFC*): When the AFC exceeds 10 follicles in each ovary, whether or not other criteria for PCO are present, much greater care is required with regard to gonadotropin administration.

AMH Level: Although there is no consensus regarding the precise level of AMH that predicts ovarian hypersensitivity to FSH, it is understood that AMH levels generally correlate with the AFC. Various assay kits may still yield inconsistent results, but a reading in excess of 5 ng/l should be taken as a warning sign.

Primary prevention consists of adjusting the management of gonadotropin administration, particularly in the choices of the stimulation protocol and of the staring dose.

8.2.3.2 Secondary Prevention

Management of an unexpected risk for OHSS that arises *during* the ovarian stimulation is possible by either by:

- *Decreasing the FSH dose*, thereby allowing only the more sensitive follicle(s) to develop, or by
- *Stopping gonadotropin administration altogether*

In a classic stimulation protocol, stopping gonadotropin administration is possible only in spontaneously ovulating patients who already have sufficient endogenous gonadotropin secretion. When the latter fails or is too erratic, follicular development stops. During a multifollicular stimulation, a "coasting" may be attempted. Typically, after gonadotropin administration has been interrupted for one or several days, and estradiol levels begin to drop, ovulation can be triggered when it reaches the safety range. This strategy may be able to rescue some IVF stimulation cycles, but the situation requires delicate management and may result in a suboptimal oocyte quality. Thus a "coasting" approach cannot be generally recommended for rescuing cycles at risk for OHSS [3]. The situation may lead to a diminished chance of success, so all options must be discussed with the patient. Furthermore, the risk of an OHSS developing nevertheless cannot be totally excluded. Therefore, it may be best to stop the cycle altogether in most cases when OHSS appears to start, and to begin another one with different parameters.

8.2.3.3 Tertiary Prevention

This approach becomes necessary when OHSS is definitely underway. The procedure involves the triggering criteria, which are not precisely defined and can vary substantially between fertility centers or even between clinicians within the same fertility setting. Although it is well established that no ideal criterion of hormone or ultrasonic measures is able to eliminate risk for OHSS, some rules and limits should nevertheless be firmly adopted in every clinical practice. The author presents here his personal criteria for each type of stimulation protocol that may be considered an adequate starting point from which each clinician may then shift according to one's own experiences and objectives.

Withdrawal from hCG in a situation recognized to be at risk for OHSS remains always the best decision, and possibly followed by contraceptive measures,. Unfortunately, making this consensual decision may conflict with a number of practical considerations, variously described as "the human factor," that result in hCG triggering nevertheless.

Among the more commonly posed reasons for continuing:

- The treatment cycle has already involved a great deal of effort and personal investment of the couple, not to mention the financial cost.
- The frustration of stopping a stimulation cycle on the heels of previously failed cycles.
- OHSS did not appear in a previous cycle that showed a comparable level of risk.
- The cycle at risk is the last of a series, and/or the undertaking of a new treatment will not be possible for some time.

These uncomfortable situations lead to impatience for the couple and some guilt for the clinician, who more or less consciously senses a responsibility for successive treatment failures. Of course, every physician has days like these, and this usually helps one understand why nearly all instances of OHSS were predictable as well as preventable.

Reduction of the hCG triggering dose: In a classical stimulation, the standard dose of 5,000 IU u-hCG or 250 µg r-hCG is in fact unnecessarily high. We and others have shown that satisfactory results may be obtained with 1,500 IU u-hCG [7]. Likewise, reducing the triggering hCG dose in a COH decreases, although it does not totally eliminate, the risk for OHSS. On the other hand, if the pregnancy rate can be maintained with a dose of 3,000 IU, chances for pregnancy may be diminished with a triggering dose of 2,500 IU or even less [8, 9]. Dose reduction may also be modulated in accordance with the patient's BMI or the estradiol levels [9, 10].

Addition of FSH to hCG: The co-administration of 450 IU rFSH with hCG may be able to lower the risk for OHSS, except in women with a low BMI. The underlying mechanism for this effect remains unresolved [11].

Substitution of LH for hCG: The principal risk for OHSS is the result of an intense, prolonged effect of hCG on the follicles and corpora lutea that does not occur with pituitary LH. Thus the use of natural LH, hLH, or rLH to trigger ovulation significantly reduces the risk for OHSS. Unfortunately this option remains unrealistic simply because of the large amount of rLH that is required and its corresponding cost [12].

Another approach, proposed by a growing number of fertility teams over the past 25 years, is to provoke an endogenous surge of FSH and LH by using a short lived GnRH agonist. There are some reports of spectacular results regarding the diminished risk for OHSS and multiple pregnancies [13]. This author has indeed observed only a few cases of twin pregnancies and/or of very modest ovarian hyperstimulation with GnRH administration in the face of a risky classic or multifollicular stimulation. A single intra-nasal or subcutaneous dose of any short acting available GnRH agonist is sufficient to trigger a maximal pituitary response, since the gonadotropin surge profile will not be greater with higher agonist doses. The compound most used at present appears to be triptorelin 0.1 mg, basically because it is packaged in seven single doses. Most other agonists are supplied in larger, more expansive packages designed for several weeks of daily doses.

Let me add a personal account at this point: More than 20 years ago I approached the French division of the concerned pharmaceutical company to request validation studies of triptorelin use as a trigger for stimulated ovulation. My motivation was a concern for patient safety that was being placed at higher risk by other triggering methods. After several discussions, the proposition failed to move forward, for two principal reasons: (1) a commercial reason, due to the relatively low price of u-hCG; and (2) a scientific reason, due to the practical and ethical difficulty at that time of conducting a double-blind prospective study comparing two groups equally at risk for OHSS. However, it would seem that randomized controlled trials should not be necessary if one can establish a clearly superior level of efficacy and safety from corroborating observational studies (see, for example, the letter by Kol drawing this analogy to proving parachute safety) [14].

Despite the absence of definitive statistical proof, the GnRH agonist approach for triggering ovulation is being adopted by ever more clinician teams who seek a "hyperstimulation-free clinic." The method is especially effective in cases of COH treated with antagonist protocols, but is of course impossible with long agonist protocols because of pituitary desensitization already created by earlier GnRH treatment. The usual triggering dose appears to be triptorelin 0.1 mg for classical stimulations, or 0.2 mg in COH antagonist protocols. Why is this higher dose preferred in COH, as no comparative studies have been conducted? Evidence suggests that the gonadotropin surge profiles provoked by both doses are identical. Undoubtedly those promoting the method for COH initially chose the 0.2 mg dosage, perhaps because higher numbers of mature follicles are available in a COH stimulation, and also because there is in fact no established risk for GnRH agonist overdosing.

On important caveat, however: whereas the method of GnRH agonist triggering extensively reduces, yet fails to eliminate, all risk for primary (early) OHSS, it is much less preventive of a secondary (late) OHSS in case of pregnancy, that can be equally serious. Management of the latter problem in COH requires a "freeze all" strategy that includes no embryo transfer.

The availability of GnRH agonist triggering as a means to minimize risk for OHSS should not be taken as encouragement for irresponsibility or carelessness. The art of managing a COH always requires a need to avoid overstimulation hazards and when a risk develops, the trigger must not be done. The unfortunate problem is that, for the variety of reasons discussed above, triggering may be done anyway. Thus, in cases recognized to be at risk for serious hyperstimulation and/or multiple pregnancy, hCG should be replaced by endogenous pituitary LH whenever possible.

8.2.3.4 Final Prevention

Even after hCG has been administered, it might still be possible to reduce the risk for OHSS, or to decrease its severity. Several approaches, although nonconsensual or not validated, have been suggested, that should not threaten a beginning pregnancy.

Intravenous administration of albumin or another large molecule such as hydroxylethyl starch (Hespan®, Hestar®). This has a high binding capacity for steroids and vasoactive compounds and diminishes their bioavailability. The substances also serve to increase colloid osmotic pressure and thus assist in maintaining plasma volume [15].

Glucocorticoids will diminish the effect of vascular endothelial growth factor (VEGF) on capillary smooth muscle, thereby reducing peripheral vasodilatation and capillary permeability [16].

Dopamine (D2) agonists that bind to capillary VEGF receptors will limit the role of VEGF in the development of hyperpermeability without compromising angiogenesis. Cabergoline is the most extensively investigated agonist, possibly because of better overall patient tolerance. Starting on the day of hCG administration, a 0.5 mg daily dose for at least one week has been shown to decrease the frequency of OHSS episodes without interfering with an imminent pregnancy [4]. Cabergoline treatment has also been shown to enhance the prevention effect for early OHSS following GnRH agonist triggering in patients with extremely high estradiol levels (>6,000 pg/ml) [17].

GnRH antagonists would appear at present to be the best early treatment for primary severe OHSS that follows a risky triggering. If all signs, clinical and ultrasound, point to a beginning OHSS, administration of 0.25 mg ganirelix sc daily for 4 days should rapidly diffuse the complication [18]. If done as part of an IVF procedure, a prolonged in vitro culture must be chosen, and an ultrasound and hormonal check-up realized on the fifth day after oocyte harvest: when there is a rising OHSS, all the embryos should be frozen for later transfer. In patients who do not show an early OHSS at this moment, continuation with a fresh transfer results in birth rates similar to those of high risk patients who do not develop severe early OHSS and who did not receive GnRH antagonist in the luteal phase [19]. This preventive effect of GnRH antagonists upon the development of OHSS seems to be mediated through a reduction of VEGF levels [20].

None of these methods is completely able to prevent the development of OHSS, inasmuch as the level of proof is weak. Furthermore, each has some potentially serious adverse effects, and must only be considered as last-chance measures.

8.2.4 Treatment of Ovarian Hyperstimulation Syndrome

Management choices for OHSS depend upon the degree of severity and must always be undertaken with great care, since any type of OHSS may suddenly worsen in case a pregnancy occurs [21].

Mild OHSS can be managed by bed rest, treatment of symptoms, and observation of weight. Problems should resolve within a few days after the onset of menses.

Moderate OHSS may require a short-term hospitalization, where a very close observation of body weight, biological parameters, and fluid input/output can be instituted. Thrombotic complications can be diminished by support stockings and administration of low molecular weight heparin.

Severe OHSS of whatever degree requires movement into intensive medical care and may require evacuation of peritoneal and sometimes pleural fluid. On the other hand, conservative management of OHSS without paracentesis has also been claimed to yield satisfactory results, along with a significant cost reduction [22].

Conclusion

Ovarian hyperstimulation, even of moderate intensity, remains a painful experience for each patient, so much so that some will abandon their quest for a pregnancy rather than risk another such incident. For this reason alone, undertaking deliberate but unjustified actions that carry a risk for development of OHSS should be strongly discouraged. Concession of the stimulation cycle remains the most appropriate, consistent decision and is always preferable over any degree of hyperstimulation.

References

1. Adashi EY, Barri P, Berkovitz R et al (2003) Infertility therapy-associated multiple pregnancies (births): an ongoing epidemic. Reprod Biomed Online 7:515–542
2. Nouri K, Haslinger P, Szabo L et al (2014) Polymorphisms of VEGF and VEGF receptors are associated with the occurrence of ovarian hyperstimulation syndrome (OHSS) – a retrospective case–control study. J Ovarian Res 7:54
3. D'Angelo A, Amso N (2002) "Coasting" (withholding gonadotropins) for prevention of ovarian hyperstimulation syndrome. Cochrane Database Syst Rev 3:CD002811
4. Soares SR (2012) Etiology of OHSS and use of dopamine agonists. Fertil Steril 97:517–522
5. Pietrowski P, Szabo L, Sator M et al (2012) Ovarian hyperstimulation syndrome is correlated with a reduction of soluble receptor protein level and a higher amount of VEGF-A. Hum Reprod 27:196–199
6. Humaidan P, Quartarolo J, Papanikolaou EG (2010) Preventing ovarian hyperstimulayion syndrome: guidance for the clinician. Fertil Steril 94:389–400
7. Emperaire JC, Parneix I, Broussin B, Ruffie A (1988) Triggering ovulation with different doses of human chorionic gonadotropin (hCG) in stimulated cycles. In: 16th world congress on fertility and sterility, Abstract O-47, p 55
8. Abdalla HI, Ah-Moye M, Brindsen P (1987) The effect of the dose of human chorionic gonadotropin and the type of gonadotropin stimulation on an *in vitro* fertilization program. Fertil Steril 48:958–963
9. Kolibianakis EM, Papanikolaou EG, Tournaye H et al (2007) Triggering final oocyte maturation using different doses of human chorionic gonadotropin: a randomized pilot study in patients with polycystic ovarian syndrome treated with gonadotropin-releasing hormone antagonist and recombinant follicle stimulating hormone. Fertil Steril 88:1382–1388
10. Chen D, Burmeister L, Goldschlag D, Rozenwaks Z (2003) Ovarian hyperstimulation syndrome: strategies for prevention. Reprod Biomed Online 7:43–49
11. Rosen MP, Meldrum DR (2012) Can FSH co-trigger prevent OHSS? Fertil Steril 97:534–535
12. The European Recombinant LH Study Group (2001) The recombinant luteinizing hormone is as effective as, but safer than, urinary human chorionic gonadotropin in inducing final follicular maturation and ovulation in *in vitro* fertilization procedures: results of a multi-center double-blind study. J Clin Endocrinol Metab 86:2607–2618
13. Emperaire JC (1994) Le déclenchement thérapeutique de l'ovulation: vers le remplacement de l'HCG par l'LH. Contra Fertil Sexual 22:459–467

14. Kol S (2006) GnRH agonist trigger: looking for the coin under the lamppost? Hum Reprod 21:1328
15. Asch RH, Ivery G, Goldman M et al (1993) The use of intravenous albumin in patients at high risk for severe ovarian hyperstimulation syndrome. Hum Reprod 8:1015–1020
16. Nauck M, Karakiulakis G, Perruchaud AP et al (1998) Corticosteroids inhibit the expression of the vascular endothelial growth factor gene in human vascular smooth muscle cells. Eur J Pharmacol 341:309–315
17. Leitao VM, Moroni RM, Seko LM et al (2014) Cabergoline for the prevention of ovarian hyperstimulation syndrome: systematic review and meta-analysis of randomized controlled trials. Fertil Steril 101:664–675
18. Lainas TG, Kolibianakis LE, Sfontouris AI et al (2012) Outpatient management of severe early OHSS by administration of GnRH antagonist in the luteal phase: an observational cohort study. Reprod Biol Endocrinol 10:69–74
19. Lainas GT, Kolibianakis ME, Sfontouris AI et al (2013) Pregnancy and neonatal outcomes following luteal GnRH antagonist administration in patients with severe OHSS. Hum Reprod 28(7):1929–1942
20. Lainas GT, Kolibianakis AM, Sfontouris IA et al (2014) Serum vascular endothelial growth factor levels following gonadotrophin-releasing hormone antagonist administration in women with severe early ovarian hyperstimulation syndrome. Hum Reprod 28:1929–1942
21. Lamazou F, Legouez A, Letouzey V (2011) Le syndrome d'hyperstimulation ovarienne: physiopathologie, facteurs de risque, prevention et prise en charge. J Gynacol Obstet Reprod 40:593–611
22. Casals G, Fábregues F, Pavesi M et al (2013) Conservative medical treatment of ovarian hyperstimulation syndrome: a single center series and cost analysis. Acta Obstet Gynecol Scand 92:686–691

9 Classic Ovulation Stimulation: Mono-, Bi-, and Paucifollicular

Classic ovulation stimulation involves three successive steps:

1. Stimulating follicular growth with a goal of producing one to three fully-developed follicles
2. Triggering ovulation to induce follicular rupture and extrusion of the oocyte(s) that have resumed meiosis and become fertilizable
3. Establishing a corpus luteum capable of sustaining implantation and development of the early embryo

It should be noted at this point that most of the effort involving protocol development have essentially concerned the stimulation step. However it is at least as important that the two other steps should progress in a harmonious way that facilitates chances for a successful pregnancy in the selected indication, be it correction of ovulation abnormalities, restoration of ovulation, improvement of cervical mucus, or preparation for an intra-uterine insemination.

9.1 Objectives

The stimulation itself should work toward two principal goals:

To mimic or adjust the normal menstrual cycle. Stimulation of monofollicular development consists of provoking or facilitating growth of one single follicle in the same manner normally accomplished by physiologic menstrual cycle, whereas a paucifollicular stimulation seeks the growth of two or three follicles. In order to mimic or alter slightly the natural cycle, one should strictly apply the rules already established by nature, i.e., to apply a strategy of gonadotropin administration that follows the basic principles of identifying an FSH threshold and window. Manipulating these parameters should attain the chosen objective, whatever the beginning situation may have been.

J.-C. Emperaire, *Ovulation Stimulation with Gonadotropins*,
DOI 10.1007/978-3-319-18654-2_9

To avoid complications: Insufficient or inadequate stimulation may result in a defective ovulatory process (e.g., abnormalities of oocyte maturation, follicular rupture, or corpus luteum function) that can paradoxically decrease the patient's chances for successful pregnancy during the treated cycle. This outcome should be considered as a true complication despite the absence of "symptoms." A succession of treatment failures make it tempting for patients to consider without due cause the more difficult road to assisted procreation, when the reality was simply a poor management of the ovarian stimulation.

Excessive stimulation is much easier to recognize because it is more symptomatic, exposing the patient to risks for ovarian hyperstimulation, multiple pregnancy, or both. The risks for these untoward results are of course greater in paucifollicular than monofollicular stimulations.

Ovarian hyperstimulation might occur only when development of the leading follicle(s) evolves in concert with numerous smaller follicles (<10 mm), a situation that can be easily discovered by ultrasound and plasma estradiol levels that rise abnormally high for one to three mature follicles.

Multiple pregnancy can only occur when a dominant and additional secondary follicles develop together, and become capable of growing and ovulating during the activity lifespan of the hCG injection that was intended to trigger only the lead follicle.

9.2 Methods of Stimulation

The difference between a successful stimulation and a defective stimulation leading to cycle cancellation has less to do with the choice of gonadotropin preparation and more to do with the administration protocol. The somewhat more simple monofollicular stimulation will be described here first, with the means for recruiting and sustaining the development of one or more additional follicles being reserved for the section on paucifollicular stimulation.

Basically, the parameters of "step-up," "step-down," or combined protocols are chosen to locate the FSH threshold, to manage the FSH window, and then to sustain appropriate follicular development so that only the optimal follicle continues to mature.

9.2.1 The Starting Dose

The prevailing consensus about an FSH threshold was first described 25 years ago by Brown and his colleagues [1], in an era prior to ultrasound technology. They also stressed the concept of inter-patient variability for this threshold, as well as more limited inter-cycle variations within the same patient. Because the ovarian follicle seems to respond to a particular level of FSH rather than to a particular administered dose, the issue is in fact how to characterize the relationship of injected dosage to resulting blood level. This is a complex multifactorial relationship that depends on severable variables:

- Existing endogenous FSH secretion that occurs in every patient, except for those rare instances of hypogonadotropic hypogonadism
- The route of administration, particularly when thick layers of subcutaneous fat create a "depot" effect at the injection site
- The volume of distribution of injected FSH that is also somewhat related to the patient's BMI
- The metabolic clearance rate of the FSH preparation that varies according to its isoform composition and degree of sialylation, and also in relation to the patient's age; these parameters all affect accumulation of hormone in plasma
- Inter-patient variations of FSH threshold related to: (a) individual physiologic parameters specific to each patient, which can account for different FSH plasma levels resulting from identical injections, and (b) variable ovarian sensitivity to FSH within each patient, which explains why patients will react differently to the same FSH level

Relationships between plasma levels and FSH threshold have been extensively investigated by Schoemaker, who monitored plasma levels daily while making very precise adjustments to dosing in order to restrict variations in plasma on the order of 1 IU/l [2]. It was found that the quantity of injected gonadotropin necessary to obtain the same plasma FSH level could vary substantially from one patient to another, but that inter- and intra-patient variations in the ovarian response to a given FSH plasma level are much smaller, save for PCO patients. While "usual" patients can be expected to show no follicular response to blood levels below 7.8 IU/l, the actual FSH threshold can vary from 6.3 to 9.8 IU/l in PCO patients with large inter-individual variations being related to differences in ovarian sensitivity.

Aside from these variations between patients, the FSH threshold and thus the starting dose are also correlated to other parameters such as patient age, AFC, AMH level, and her BMI. Several attempts for predicting the best FSH starting dose have been proposed: for example, Frieseleben's algorithm that takes into account only the patient's AFC and weight [3]. However, these are only probabilities, and for an initial stimulation cycle it seems preferable to lean toward a lower dose if only because an insufficient dosage is easier to handle than an excessive one.

9.2.2 Selecting a Protocol

Schoemaker's study also confirms that a minimal increase of FSH, as low as 1 IU/L above the threshold, may lead to multifollicular development. This finding illustrates two main basic principles:

- The increment of administered gonadotropin doses must remain small, so that plasma FSH levels do not rise too rapidly. There is indeed a narrow range between

the dose which elicits no response, even if administered indefinitely, and the dose responsible for multifollicular development. This dose range may not exceed 25–37.5 IU, and perhaps less.
- The increment of FSH doses must remain progressive, as it takes 4–6 days for plasma hormone levels to stabilize, and also because the follicular recruitment period may spread over 5–15 days. This explains why FSH may be administered in three different types of protocol.

9.2.2.1 The "Step-Up" Protocols

Definitions of the protocols for gonadotropin administration began in the mid-1960s, when monitoring by measuring levels of urinary estrogens became available. The earlier stimulation method originally proposed by Crooke, that utilized very high single dosing or a fractionated 3-dose process was abandoned for one of two "step-up" designs [4]:

- A Lunenfeld-Rabau proposal that each dose increment should be 75 IU (one HMG vial)
- A proposal by Brown that increments should not increase over the previous dose by more than one-third

The Israeli protocol continues as the more frequently used, although many Australian clinicians have held strongly to Brown's ideas.

9.2.3 The Standard Step Up Protocol

Basically because of its simplicity, this remains the most widely used protocol, particularly for spontaneously ovulating women. The fundamental approach begins with a daily FSH dose of 50–75 IU, with the first monitoring conducted after 5–7 days of administration. If no mature follicle is detected, there are three possible situations (Fig. 9.1):

A beginning follicular response, evidenced by the appearance at ultrasound of a follicle of at least 10 mm diameter plus a concomitant rise of plasma estradiol. In this case the stimulation should continue with the same FSH dose, and a second evaluation should be scheduled for 2–3 days later. Experience has shown that the starting dose can be continued throughout the complete stimulation cycle in most cases.

Absent follicular response: the absence of visual evidence of any developing follicles suggests that the FSH threshold has not been reached. The dose should be increased by 50 or 100 % in line with the plasma estradiol profile. It there is still no response after another 5–7 days, the FSH dose may be increased once or twice more, but if no development ensues, it is preferable to stop the present stimulation cycle and undertake a new cycle with a higher starting dose.

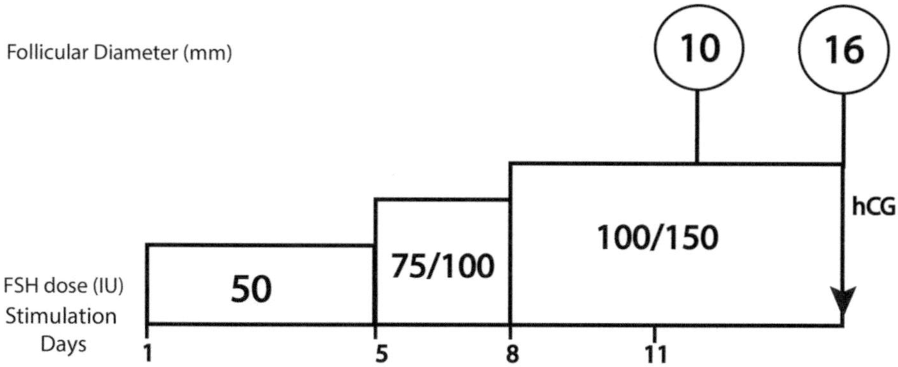

Fig. 9.1 Step-up standard protocol

A plurifollicular response accompanied by rapidly rising estradiol levels. This indicates that the FSH threshold has been overcome. One might consider beginning a "step down" approach, but it may also be prudent to stop the present cycle and undertake a new stimulation cycle using a lower starting dose of FSH, a step-up low dose protocol, or both.

The theoretical drawback of these traditional step-up protocols is that they often move rather distant from the principles of a natural cycle, nevertheless requiring a careful monitoring. On the other hand, this design offers an advantage of dose adaptations over short periods of time. In addition, it is fairly simple to manage, particularly with clinicians who are still relatively inexperienced with ovarian stimulation protocols. Further, the design is relatively simple for patients to follow. Only one or two monitoring controls are required per cycle, and indeed the strategy is quite effective in most spontaneously ovulating women.

9.2.4 The Step-Up Low Dose Protocol

Because of persistent risks for multifollicular development in PCO patients, occurring despite using urinary FSH in a standard step-up protocol, Siebel was led to define the principles for a low dose treatment strategy. It should be pointed out that his initial proposal was simply to reverse the FSH/LH ratio of the injections by administrating "pure" FSH [5]. Polson deserves credit for revisiting the concept of an FSH threshold by folding in an initial administration of low FSH doses [6]. The latter step actually adopted Brown's initial recommendations for a more progressive increase in the FSH doses, because he had noted that in certain patients, an increment of only 10–30 % was sufficient to move from no response to a plurifollicular reaction. Without the help of ultrasound, this author proposed to start stimulations at 100 IU FSH for 5 days, and if no follicular response were detected, to increase this daily dose by 30 % every 5 days until a response appears. This final level of dosing is then continued until ovulation is triggered [1].

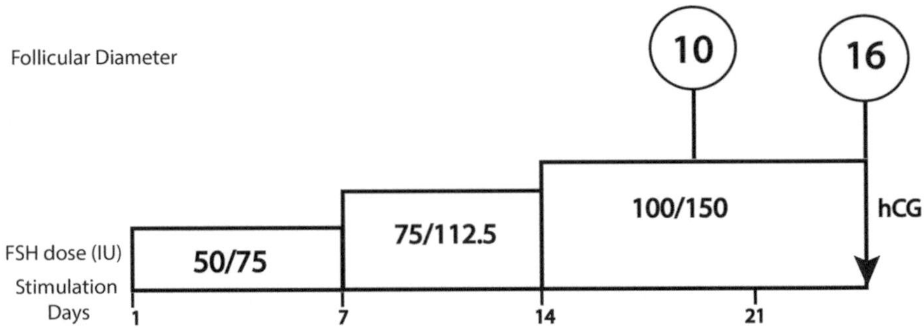

Fig. 9.2 Step-up low-dose protocol

In practice, the low-dose step-up protocols usually begin with 50–75 IU FSH daily for 7 days (Fig. 9.2). If a 10 mm diameter follicle appears by this point, the same dose is maintained until the triggering criteria are met. If there is no follicular response after 7 days of stimulation, the dose is increased by *half* the initial dose for another 7 days, and so on. When a follicular response does appear, this dose is maintained until ovulation is triggered.

In case of an excessive response, it is still possible to diminish the FSH dose, or to stop the treatment cycle altogether, and start another one with a lower initial dose, and/or to proceed with only 25 % increments of the initial dose. If hyper-responsive difficulties persist, move to an even lower dose protocol.

The more physiologic design of this step-up low-dose protocol avoids many hyper-responses, and monitoring is not more demanding. For this reason the protocol has progressively replaced the standard step up in non ovulatory patients.

9.2.5 The Step Up Chronic Low-Dose Protocol

This design begins in similar fashion to the low dose protocol by starting with 50–75 IU FSH for 7 days. If a response does not appear, the same dose is maintained for another 7 days, in contrast to the low dose protocol, because this treatment interval is closer to the recruitment duration that may run between 5 and 15 days (Fig. 9.3).

If no response appears after 14 days, then the FSH dose is increased by half of the initial dose for another 7 days, and then increased similarly at weekly intervals, as with the low-dose protocol. When a follicular response finally occurs, the FSH dose remains unchanged until ovulation triggering.

If no response is observed after 35 days of stimulation, the cycle should be abandoned, and the next one initiated at 150 % of the previous starting dose. On the other hand, if the response becomes excessive, the stimulation cycle must be halted and the next treatment cycle begun with a lower starting dose of FSH.

The low-dose and chronic low-dose step-up protocols yield comparable results in anovulatory patients [7]. In contrast to the standard step-up protocol, the

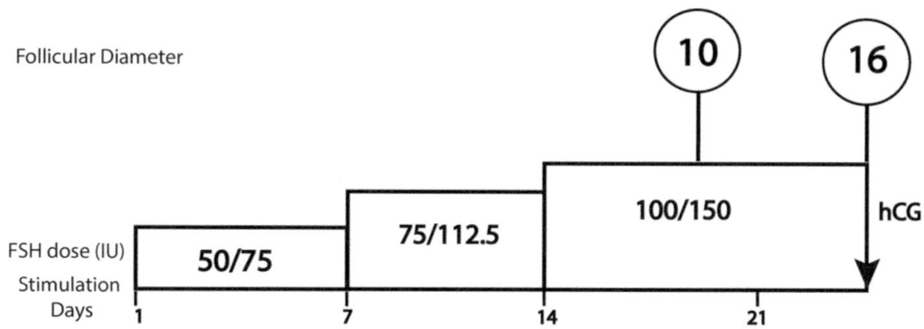

Fig. 9.3 Step-up chronic low-dose protocol

step-up low-dose designs represent a true advance for some PCO patients because they combine a high rate monofollicular cycles and of successful pregnancy together with a substantial reduction of risks for multiple pregnancy and/or OHHS. On the other hand, a drawback to this protocol is the need for continuous monitoring during stimulation that may potentially go on for several weeks. This can lead to problems of feasibility or compliance, although only some 10 % of patients appear to discontinue treatment because of lack of ovarian response after 35 days of stimulation. To avoid these overly lengthy stimulation phases, one may consider starting a new cycle with a slightly higher FSH dose than the dose level that reached the FSH threshold in the previous cycle, even if that leads to a decreased dose later on. On the other hand, if the chronic low-dose level remains too high, it is still possible to decrease the starting dose and/or the dose increment (e.g., by one-fourth of the initial dose), thereby creating a sort of step-up, chronic, ultra-low dose protocol.

All the step-up protocols do vary somewhat from the physiologic spontaneous menstrual cycle. While they usually reach the FSH threshold in a more or less progressive fashion, they also maintain this elevated dose throughout the whole stimulation period. In a normal physiologic cycle, levels of FSH elevate rapidly during the first few cycle days, and then decline throughout the remainder of the follicular phase. Maintaining a dose regimen that achieves an FSH plasma level higher than the threshold may hold the FSH window open for recruitment of additional follicles, thus producing a plurifollicular response. Repeated daily administration of a fixed FSH dose will cause an over-abundance of hormone in plasma by the end of the stimulation phase. All of these potential drawbacks are taken into account in the design of the step-down protocols.

9.2.5.1 The Step-Down Protocol

This protocol initially designed by Mizunuma et al. was later extensively studied and refined by Fauser et al. [8, 9]. It was initially confirmed that the early rise of FSH in normal menstrual cycles reached a mean of 6 IU/l on cycle day 5, with a variance factor of 2.5 between women. Hormone levels were then observed to diminish by 0.5 IU/l per day to a mean nadir of 2.9 IU/l on cycle day 13. They also reported that the first detectable rise of the plasma estradiol coincides with the ultrasound appearance of a 9–10 mm diameter structure, namely the emerging dominant follicle.

The principle of the step down protocol is to start the stimulation with an FSH dose tailored to overcome the FSH threshold so that several of the most sensitive elements of the ovarian follicular pool begin to grow. Once the dominant follicle has appeared, the daily FSH dose is then progressively *reduced* so that only the most sensitive follicle continues to develop (Fig. 9.4).

In practice the stimulation sequence begins with 150 IU FSH daily for 5 days:

- If monitoring shows the beginning of an ovarian response, the FSH dose is decreased by a fourth every 3 days until a minimum of 75 IU, and this dose is maintained until ovulation triggering.
- If there is no ovarian response after 5 days of stimulation, the daily dose is increased by 37.5 IU every 5 days, for a maximum of two additional increases.
- If there is still no ovarian response after 15 days of stimulation, the cycle should be halted, and the next treatment cycle should start with a dose of 187.5 IU (125 % of the previous starting dose).

This protocol, while attractive in theory, may in fact be somewhat difficult to manage:

For one thing, the precise moment for reducing the FSH dose, marked by the appearance of a 9–10 mm follicle together with an estrogenic response, is not always easy to recognize, and problems of interpretation may occur. Diminishing the FSH dose too early might lead to an irreversible follicular atresia, and reducing the dose too late may lead to plurifollicular stimulation, two opposing causes leading to the same outcome, i.e., abandoning the treatment cycle.

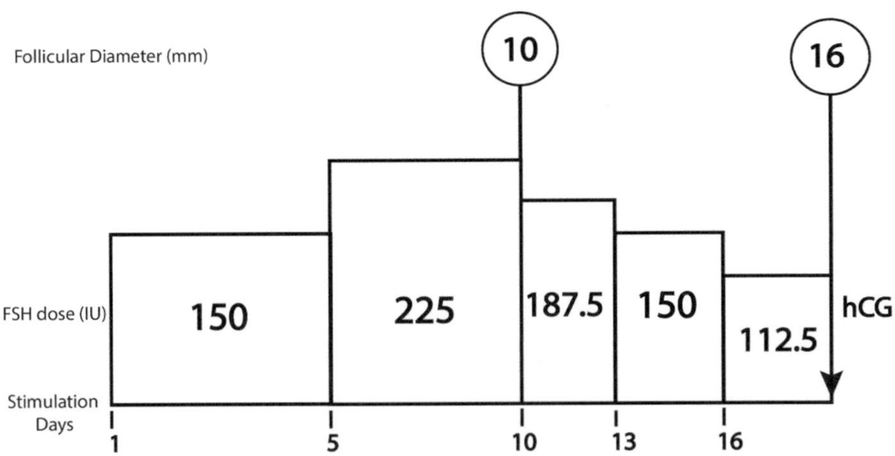

Fig. 9.4 Step-down protocol

Another problem is that the proposed starting dose of 150 IU FSH is arbitrary and does not take into account the FSH threshold of each patient. 150 IU may be quite excessive for some patients, and provoke a plurifollicular development that the successive dose reductions may not be able to control. This again can lead to having to stop the cycle and start another one at 50 % of the previous starting dose.

9.2.6 Step-Up and Step-Down (Sequential) Protocol

This approach combining the step-up and step-down protocols was first made by JN Hughes, in order to benefit from the advantages of each. The stimulation begins similarly to a step-up low-dose protocol, so that the FSH dose does not overcome ovarian sensitivity. Once the dominant follicle is recognized, the same dose is maintained for a few days, and then is decreased in order to prevent development of secondary and tertiary follicles. This secondary reduction in the FSH dose is thus delayed, in contrast to the regular step-down protocol [10].

Specifically, the sequential protocol should be conducted as follows (Fig. 9.5):

- Begin stimulation with a 50–75 IU FSH dose for 6–7 days, then increase by half of the starting dose (25–37.5 IU) at intervals of the same duration until a 9–10 mm diameter follicle appears
- Maintain the same FSH dose until the dominant follicle reaches the empirically chosen diameter of 14 mm
- Reduce the FSH dose by half and maintain this level until the ovulation is triggered

This attractive protocol, like the step-down protocol, may also encounter problems, mainly being able to recognize with certainty the crucial moment when the FSH dose should be reduced.

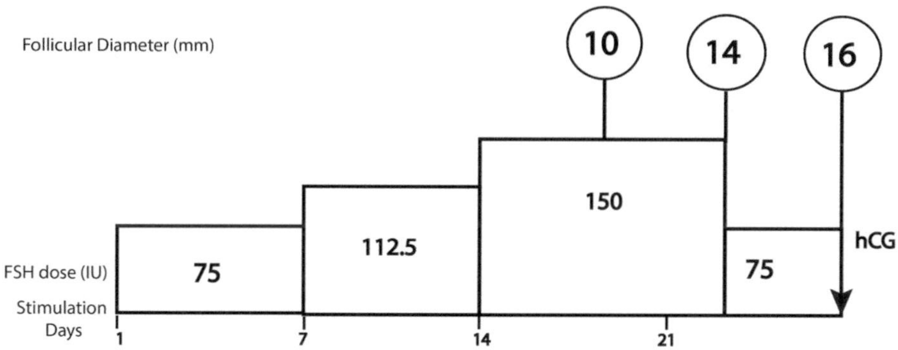

Fig. 9.5 Sequential step-up/step-down protocol

9.2.7 Summary

Clinicians finally have at hand a variety of therapeutic plans that should resolve every sort of challenging problem posed by the stimulation process.

Step-up protocols continue to be the most widely used to initial trials, and remain the standard approach for ovulatory women. On the other hand, nonovulatory patients should be initially started with a low-dose schedule.

Step-down and sequential protocols share the same difficulties regarding the decision point for reducing the FSH dose. More experience may be necessary before undertaking these protocols because they are more operator-dependent as well as harder to reproduce. They are especially tailored for the very few patients who are hypersensitive to FSH, especially following failures with low dose and ultra low dose protocols. Furthermore, abandonment of several consecutive stimulation cycles after many daily injections and monitoring controls may lead even the most dedicated patient to relinquish her treatment.

9.3 Stimulation Monitoring

Monitoring must be conducted using both hormonal and ultrasound parameters. Conventional 2D ultrasound is quite adequate for measuring the mean diameter of one or several follicles. The plasma estradiol assay is mandatory, as estradiol production reaches a maximum 6 h after FSH administration and is maintained at this level for at least 24 h [11]; it also helps to distinguish a functional follicle from a follicular cyst. A progesterone assay is useful for detection of a possible premature luteinization, and the LH assay is necessary to locate the best moment for a single intercourse or insemination.

There are three basic principles for adapting FSH doses to the ovarian response. All are related to the dynamics of estradiol levels and ultrasound data, and all are fairly intangible:

- *Decrease* the FSH dose when estradiol increases faster than follicular growth
- *Maintain* the same FSH dose when the estradiol rise and follicular growth are at the same rate
- *Increase* the FSH dose when the estradiol level lags behind follicular growth; when this type of response repeats itself on the next cycle, consider to add LH to FSH administration

These principles underlie the reason why protocols that rely only on ultrasound data are merely indicative and incomplete. At similar ultrasound readings, measures of estradiol patterns will lead to different clinical decisions.

For example, in cases of discrepancy between ultrasound evaluation and estrogen responses:

- A beginning estrogen response without a recognizable ultrasound reaction may lead to a decision to delay the FSH dose increase
- A beginning ultrasound response with no sign of an estradiol rise may lead to increasing the FSH dose sooner than originally scheduled.

Finally, the rhythm and number of monitoring controls should of course be suited to the selected protocol, and also to the patient's possibilities. While it remains true that conducting more frequent controls brings more precision to the monitoring process, the rules should sometimes be softened, and whenever possible consider the situation, sensibility, and availability of each patient.

References

1. Brown JB (1978) Pituitary control of ovarian function: concepts derived from gonadotropin therapy. Aust N Z J Obstet Gynaecol 18:47–54
2. Schoemaker J, Van Weissenbruch MM, Van Der Meer M (1993) New approaches with the FSH threshold principle in polycystic ovary syndrome. Ann N Y Acad Sci 687:296–300
3. Freiseleben NC, Lossi K, Bogstad J et al (2008) Predictors of ovarian response in intrauterine insemination patients and development of a dosage normogram. Reprod Biomed Online 17:632–641
4. Crooke AC (1964) The clinical effects of pituitary and urinary gonadotropins. Proc R Soc Med 57:111–114
5. Siebel MM, Kamrava M, Mac Ardle C, Trevor ML (1984) Treatment of polycystic ovary disease with chronic low dose follicle-stimulating hormone: biochemical changes and ultrasound correlations. Int J Fertil 29:39–43
6. Polson DW, Mason HD, Saldahna MA, Franks S (1987) Ovulation of a single dominant follicle during treatment with low dose pulsatile follicle stimulating hormone in women with polycystic ovary syndrome. Clin Endocrinol 26:205–212
7. Serour GI, Aboulghar M, Al Bahar A et al (2014) Phase IV, open label, randomized study of low-dose recombinant human follicle stimulating hormone protocols for ovulation induction. Reprod Biol Endocrinol 12:52–62
8. Mizunuma H, Takagi T, Yamada K et al (1991) Ovulation induction by step down administration of purified urinary follicle-stimulating hormone in patients with polycystic ovarian syndrome. Fertil Steril 55:1195–1196
9. Fauser BC, De Jong FH (1993) Gonadotropins in polycystic ovarian syndrome. Ann N Y Acad Sci 687:150–161
10. Hugues JN, Cedrin-Durnein I, Avril C et al (1996) Sequential step-up and step-down regimen: an alternative method for ovulation induction with follicle-stimulation hormone in polycystic ovarian syndrome. Hum Reprod 11:2581–2584
11. Coffler MJ, Patel K, Dahan MH et al (2014) Evidence for abnormal granulosa cell responsiveness to follicle stimulating hormone in women with polycystic ovary syndrome. J Clin Endocrinol Metab 88:1742–1747

10 Stimulation in the Ovulating Patient

In a spontaneously ovulating patient, the classic stimulation protocol can be used for several purposes:

- *A monofollicular stimulation* that is intended to mimic closely the normal physiologic cycle. It is mandatory to begin with this protocol in ovulating younger patients under age 35, those with a low BMI, in patients who have been infertile for less than 3 years, and also in preparation for an intrauterine insemination (IUI) in cases of infertility of cervical origin or when using donor sperm.
- *A bifollicular stimulation* of course includes the risk for multiple pregnancy. While the possibility of a twin pregnancy may usually be acceptable in a couple that has been infertile for several years, any multiple pregnancy can become a hazardous situation with an uncertain prognosis. This sort of risk should only be undertaken when one anticipates a clear benefit from having an extra oocyte, whether for intercourse or insemination, and to compensate for certain fertility challenges such as an altered ovarian reserve, in a patient of advanced age or with a structural pelvic abnormality (e.g., a single fallopian tube, or mild endometriosis), or in case of a suboptimal sperm quality, or with an idiopathic infertility.
- *A paucifollicular stimulation.* Ovulation in the presence or three or more mature follicles is too great a risk to be undertaken, except possibly in a very select population of patients over 40 years of age, who have been fully informed of potential risks, and only after several unsuccessful bifollicular stimulation cycles.

J.-C. Emperaire, *Ovulation Stimulation with Gonadotropins*,
DOI 10.1007/978-3-319-18654-2_10

10.1 Monofollicular Stimulation

10.1.1 Indications in a Spontaneously Ovulating Woman

Mild ovulatory disorders (*dysovulation*), which typically involve a premature or delayed follicular maturation (dysmaturation), cervical mucus insufficiency, luteal phase deficiencies secondary to an ovulatory dysfunction, or an inadequate endogenous gonadotropin surge. Stimulation may also be indicated for a patient who appears to be ovulating normally but simply does not conceive. Adding FSH increases estradiol secretion and in turn optimizes the cervical mucus and endometrial development. hCG administration then ensures adequate luteinization and supports the early luteal phase.

With programmed intercourse, in the case of spontaneous inadequate cervical mucus but with a good post-coital test on estradiol treatment.

In preparation for an intrauterine insemination, in one of several situations:

- When using donor insemination in young patients, without other recognized factors, and who failed to conceive after 2 or 3 attempts with spontaneous ovulation
- In cases of infertility suspected to be due to cervical factors, or having a negative post-coital test, either as first line treatment or in patients without other recognized subfertility factors who have failed to conceive after 2 or 3 attempts with classic stimulation
- In situations of oligo-astheno-teratospermia with a recovery of at least 1 million motile spermatozoa
- After 4–6 failed classic stimulation cycles with programmed intercourse, prior to moving toward trials of IVF

In spontaneously ovulating women, even those ovulating inadequately, the aim of the stimulation is to correct a pre-existing ovulatory process. These patients do have pulsatile gonadotropin secretion and an intact feedback interaction between the follicle and the hypothalamic-pituitary axis. The addition of exogenous gonadotropins merely adjusts or stabilizes an already functioning process to a more satisfactory manner. This is the simplest type of stimulation.

10.1.2 Choosing a Gonadotropin

In a patient who spontaneously ovulates, endogenous LH secretion is presumably sufficient, thus the stimulation can be conducted with FSH only. Addition of LH does not provide any specific benefit unless plasma sampling does reveal a possible insufficiency. Any of the preparations of FSH or FSH+LH may be administered, with the caution that reconstituted lyophilized urinary extracts are more difficult to divide with accuracy and much may be wasted.

10.1.3 Choosing a Protocol

Because the treatment objective is to sustain development of a follicle that has already been selected, the stimulation should not begin earlier than the sixth or seventh cycle day, when this selection has just occurred. It is important to administer gonadotropin after the FSH window has closed, to support growth of the sole dominant follicle and not others. In case of an early follicular dysmaturation, treatment should begin earlier, on cycle day 5. The step-up standard protocol is perfectly designed for this purpose, and should be the first-line strategy for adequate stimulation in most patients. Incremental increases of gonadotropin dosage may be adjusted up to less than 100 % of the initial dose. Presence of multifollicular ovaries may lead to decreasing the starting dose, or to choosing a step-up low-dose protocol that should be considered anyway if the standard step-up treatment has resulted in an excessive response.

10.1.4 Doses of FSH

The starting dose should remain low, e.g., 50–75 IU daily. This may prove insufficient in patients with a higher BMI or in those older than their late 30s. But one cannot be certain. *It is easier to increase an insufficient dose than to manage an excessive dose*. Furthermore, higher doses might support growth of secondary follicles during the recruitment phase, and result in a pauci- or multifollicular cycle. Careful observation of the ovarian response during the first stimulation cycle will of course help manage a subsequent cycle.

10.1.5 Duration of Stimulation

The initial period of stimulation lasts 5–7 days. Five days should be sufficient to balance exogenously administered gonadotropins with endogenous pituitary secretion that should together provoke a detectable effect on follicular growth. Seven days' administration could delay the initial monitoring to cycle day 13–14, which may be too late. The first monitoring evaluation should ideally be conducted on the 11th or 12th cycle day. A second evaluation might be indicated after 2–4 additional days of treatment, depending upon results from ultrasound and hormone measures.

10.1.6 Expected Outcomes

The initial monitoring will most likely show one of the following (Table 10.1):

- A single mature follicle with a mean diameter >16 mm, plasma estradiol <350 pg/ml, and the absence of other follicles >12 mm in diameter. In this situation, hCG may be administered, with an insignificant risk for multiple pregnancy. If the mature follicle's mean diameter is borderline (15–16 mm), ovulation may be postponed until after one more day of FSH administration, without need for another monitoring visit.

- One follicle with a mean diameter >16 mm, together with secondary 13–15 mm follicles, and an estradiol level under 800 pg/ml. In this case the stimulation cycle has become paucifollicular. Administration of hCG may result in a multiple pregnancy, and this possibility should be discussed with the patient. The risk may be significantly reduced, although not totally eliminated, by triggering ovulation with a GnRH agonist. If it is decided to stop the stimulation cycle without triggering ovulation, contraceptive measures should be undertaken because spontaneous ovulation may nevertheless occur.

Table 10.1 Managing the standard step-up protocol for a mono-follicular stimulation; possible scenarios after administration of 50–75 IU FSH for 5 days (see StimXpert)

					1foll>16 ⊕	
FD mm	< 9.9	10 - 12.9	13 - 14.9	15 - 16	0 foll>12	n foll>12
E2 pg/ml						
>500	S (4)	S (4)	2	1	S (1)	S (1) (2)
250 - 500	4	3	2	1	hCG	
150 - 250	3	3	2	1	hCG	
75-150	4	3	2	1	hCG	
<75	4	3	2	1 / S (3)	S (3)	

↑ **FSH** 50 -75 IU x 5 days

Key	% of the starting dose
S STOP	
+100%	
+50%	
0%	
-50%	
0%	

- Several follicles >16 mm diameter. Administration of hCG brings a high risk for multiple pregnancy in this situation. It may also provoke an early ovarian hyperstimulation when numerous secondary follicles are present and/or plasma estradiol exceeds 800 pg/ml. hCG must not be administered in this situation, and contraceptive measures are strongly indicated. Triggering ovulation with a GnRH agonist in order to reduce the risk of hyperstimulation and multiple pregnancy may be considered, but it still may not prevent a late hyperstimulation.
- The dominant follicle is <14 mm diameter. FSH administration must continue with another evaluation made 2 or 3 days later, depending on the size of the follicle, which may grow 1.5–3 mm a day. The continued dose level of FSH should be reevaluated according to the number of growing follicles and the observed estradiol level:
  - Maintain the same dosage when $150 < E_2 < 250$ pg/ml
  - Reduce the dosage when $E_2 > 250$ pg/ml or when several other follicles are growing, so that only the most sensitive one continues to develop
  - Increase the FSH dose when $E_2 < 100$ pg/ml

The optimal time for a single intercourse would be the day after hCG or GnRH agonist administration (shortly before ovulation) so that the spermatozoa have already reached the fecundation site. Intercourse on the same day of hCG, or 2 days later, may also be effective.

This table illustrates the types of decisions that should be made with various combinations of follicular response (FD mm, *top row*) and plasma estradiol (E_2 pg/ml, *left side column*)
Within each box, The *Circle Number* indicates the optimal number of days to continue stimulation, if triggering criteria have not yet been met after 5 days of stimulation. The *Circle Color* indicates the suggested percentage change for FSH dosing in relation to the previous (starting) dose. A *White Circle* with S indicates the cycle should be stopped or abandoned with no further stimulation. Boxes with HCG identify the follicle+estrogen criteria that permit ovulation triggering. Boxes with a number in parentheses refer to 1 of 4 footnotes listed below.
When a patient is unable to come in for assessment after the indicated number of days, it remains possible to conduct the monitor one day earlier or later, possibly including a change of the FSH dose
The number of estradiol ranges has been purposely limited in order to simplify the table's construction, and should be considered as approximate when interpretations are made. In particular, when values are close to the indicated upper or lower value of E_2 within a range, the clinical decision should consider options indicated for the adjacent hormone level
Footnotes
1. Triggering with a short-acting GnRH agonist instead of hCG can significantly reduce, but will not eliminate, the risk for OHSS; additional luteal support is then mandatory
2. Triggering with a short-acting GnRH agonist instead of hCG can significantly reduce, but will not eliminate, the risk for multiple pregnancy; additional luteal support is then mandatory
3. Follicular growth that progresses faster than the rise of plasma estradiol levels may be related to an insufficient LH effect; in this case it is better to repeat the stimulation with an FSH preparation that includes LH
4. Caution: Risks for OHSS appear and increase when the plasma estradiol level reaches and surpasses 800 pg/ml

In this population of spontaneously ovulating patients, a single monitoring control is sufficient in about half of the cycles; a second evaluation becomes necessary in an additional 35 %. Three or more evaluations will be required in the remaining 15 % of patients, before the moment of triggering.

The criterion of triggering ovulation in the presence of a single follicle ≥16 mm and no other ones >12 mm would seem not to be entirely adequate because, even when strictly adhered to, a twin pregnancy results 5–10 % of the time. Except in situations when only one ovary is clearly visualized with ultrasound, there are two complementary explanations for this paradox:

Secondary follicles: 15–25 % of multiple pregnancies result when there is more than one follicle between 11 and 15 mm diameter at the time hCG is administered [1]. It is thus mandatory to take all of the smaller follicles into careful account. A single follicle of only 12 mm diameter may produce a 7.1 % pregnancy rate [2]. On the other hand, the pregnancy has every chance to remain single when no follicle aside from the mature one is >11 mm.

Duration of the hCG activity: Whereas the endogenous gonadotropin surge is some 48–54 h duration, the effect of injected hCG lasts for several days. Thus a secondary follicle may continue to grow and reach sufficient maturity to ovulate during this period of time. Its growth may indeed be stimulated by the LH-like effect of hCG at the end of the follicular phase.

hCG triggering continues to be used even in the presence of well-recognized risks for multiparous pregnancy because of a "Human Factor." For example, when two 15 mm follicles are observed on the fourth stimulation cycle, despite the utmost care to control development, or after a cycle had to be stopped for the same type of reason, or when monofollicular cycles fail to produce a pregnancy, the patient (and her clinician as well) can grow impatient.

Plasma estradiol levels are also important, and should run 150–250 pg/ml for a single mature follicle. However, smaller follicles (<11 mm) provide some estrogen secretion as well. Nevertheless, levels should remain under 800 pg/ml with a single mature follicle on a normofollicular ovary in order to avoid the early risk of OHSS.

10.1.7 Providing Luteal Support

It has never been clearly established that supplementing the post-ovulatory phase with progesterone is useful in the spontaneously ovulatory patient. Indeed a harmonious follicular development under FSH that produces a single complete follicle, then followed by an hCG trigger, can be expected to result in an adequate luteal gland providing a normal 12–14 day luteal phase. Nevertheless, caution advises one to check on both the luteal phase duration and plasma progesterone levels, which should exceed 10 ng/ml by 7–9 days post-hCG. When these criteria are not met, it is best to sustain the luteal phase with 20 mg oral retroprogesterone, 200 mg vaginal micronized progesterone, or 90 mg of 8 % vaginal progesterone gel. Treatment should start *not less than* 72 h after hCG administration in order not to impair the quality of cervical mucus. Clearly a much better way is to build a more adequate corpus luteum through a more efficient stimulation of granulosa cells.

10.1.7.1 If the First Stimulation Cycle Fails

It is possible to undertake another cycle without delay, if a preliminary ultrasound evaluation establishes the absence of residual transonic structures. A persistent follicle of less than 20 mm diameter may be tolerated, but it should be located with precision so that it will not be confused as a newly mature or pre-mature follicle. If a functional cyst of >20 mm is identified, it is better to postpone an FSH administration that would potentially stimulate its further development. Allow a month to pass, or alternatively administer 5 mg oral nomegestrol acetate for 20 days if the cyst is even larger. Stimulation may then be started on the next cycle providing the structure has disappeared.

The FSH dose should certainly be reevaluated with respect to the situations that occurred during the previous treatment cycle. Careful monitoring of each cycle is always mandatory because ovarian responses may vary from one cycle to another. Different responses are possible even when the same gonadotropin dose is administered to the same patient, and even when the patient has a history of regular responses during previous cycles. Monitoring remains mandatory even when the stimulation is conducted with only a few spaced out FSH injections given during the follicular phase of a spontaneously ovulating patient; this type of stimulation, often designed for the benefit of reducing monitoring constraints, is nevertheless incapable of ensuring an adequate stimulation and at the same time of avoiding all complications.

10.1.8 Number of Trials

Ideally, an efficient treatment in an infertile patient should restore the same chances for pregnancy as in a normally fertile woman of the same age. Because these chances approximate 20–25 % in normal younger women under optimal conditions, one should allow some time to set the appropriate limits. A stimulation program of this type should yield a satisfactory result within a maximum of 6 cycles, but every program is at risk of compression because of a couples' weariness or impatience. Realistically, for couples or patients past the age of 35, the plan may be restricted to three or four cycles, when success is most likely.

10.2 Bifollicular Stimulation

In order to increase the chances for pregnancy in a spontaneously ovulating patient, it may be appropriate to consider promotion of a second mature follicle, for various reasons:

- To compensate for another subfertility factor in addition to impaired ovulation, such as: suboptimal sperm parameters, a patient older than age 38, or presence of a pelvic abnormality, e.g., a single patent Fallopian tube or grade I–II endometriosis
- In certain instances of idiopathic infertility in the presence of a positive post-coital test

Growth of two follicles is managed by precise FSH administration. Bringing two follicles to maturity simultaneously requires careful management between two potential pitfalls [3, 4]:

- Recruiting and bringing to full maturity one additional follicle without provoking a multifollicular development
- Avoiding a twin pregnancy; that becomes a less critical risk with advancing age

Basically, it is possible to recruit an additional follicle and bring it to maturity by stretching one or both of two cardinal rules of monofollicular stimulation, namely, the moment of the cycle when stimulation is begun, and the FSH dose.

FSH administration can be started during the follicular recruitment period, i.e., earlier than the sixth day of the cycle. Building an early rise of FSH by starting on CD 3 enables plasma levels to reach the sensitivity threshold of the two most sensitive follicles, and it then supports their additional growth by disrupting the mechanisms for selection and dominance. Dosing should remain low (50–75 IU) in order to stay below the sensitivity threshold of more than two follicles.

Alternatively, FSH administration can be started a bit later, on the sixth or seventh CD, in order to delay the rise of FSH levels and "rescue" one additional follicle that was destined for atresia. In this instance a higher FSH dose (75–125 IU) should be used to provide sufficient support for development of this additional follicle by preventing the FSH window from closing. However, the enhanced dosing must not be allowed to initiate growth of any more new follicles.

These manipulations of cardinal rules were illustrated by the work of Cedrin-Durnerin, et al. [5]. With a continuous daily dose of 112 IU rFSH beginning on CD 2–3, they observed development of three to four follicles in excess of 14 mm diameter, whereas only two such follicles were recruited when the same administration was started on CD 7. This result confirmed the value of lower dose levels when beginning administration earlier in the cycle.

10.2.1 Other Suitable Protocols for a Bifollicular Stimulation

- Administration of double-sized doses of FSH (e.g., 150 IU) on alternate days (CD 4, 6 and 8), with the initial monitoring made on CD 9
- A combination of oral clomiphene, 50–100 mg for 5 days starting on CD 3, followed by a single dose of 75 or 150 IU FSH on CD 9, and the first monitoring control performed on CD 11

10.2.2 Practical Considerations

For the initial stimulation cycle in a patient whose response to FSH administration is still unknown, it is best to begin with conservative dosing of 50 or 75 IU if starting on CD 3–4, or 75–125 IU when starting on CD 6–7. Both may be adjusted for the patient's age and BMI.

At the end of the fifth day of stimulation, one of four situations is likely to appear (Table 10.2):

- Two follicles >16 mm diameter are present without secondary follicles >12 mm, and estradiol is less than 800 pg/ml. The objectives for a bifollicular cycle have been met, and the hCG trigger can be safely administered.
- More than two follicles >16 mm diameter and/or an estradiol level >800 pg/ml. In this situation administration of hCG is liable to result in a multiple pregnancy, an ovarian hyperstimulation or both. Therefore, only a GnRH agonist should be used to trigger ovulation, with the reservations previously mentioned. Otherwise, the cycle should be aborted altogether with institution of contraceptive measures.
- Only one follicle appears that is larger than 16 mm diameter, estradiol is <500 pg/ml and there are no secondary follicles greater than 12 mm diameter. The basic objectives for a bifollicular cycle may not be reached in this case. One may choose to terminate the cycle and start over, or to continue with FSH administration together with a GnRH antagonist, in the hope of growing a second mature follicle while ovulation of the larger one is being prevented by the antagonist.
- A single follicle is >16 mm diameter is found, secondary follicles are 13–15 mm diameter, or the one dominant follicle does not exceed 15 mm diameter, and estradiol level is below 500 pg/ml. Stimulation must continue with the next monitoring assessment taken 2–3 days later. The dose level of FSH should be reevaluated with respect to the number of growing follicles and the levels of plasma estradiol, as described earlier (Fig. 10.1):
  - FSH dose should remain unchanged when estradiol is between 250 and 500 pg/ml.
  - The dose should be reduced when estradiol is greater than 500 pg/ml or when more than two follicles are growing, so that only the most sensitive ones resume development.
  - The dose should be increased when $E_2 < 250$ pg/ml.

10.2.3 Complications

Complications are definitely more prone to occur in a bifollicular stimulation than with a monofollicular treatment:

Risk for multiple pregnancy: This risk, most often for twins, is very real even when the number of potentially fertilizable oocytes was increased simply to offset other subfertility factors within the couple, or in case of an idiopathic infertility.

Table 10.2 Managing the standard step-up protocol for a bi-follicular stimulation; possible scenarios after administration of 50–125 IU FSH for 5 days (see StimXpert)

FD mm	< 9.9	10 - 12.9	13 - 14.9	15 - 16	1foll>16 ⊕ 1-2foll>12	2foll>16 ⊕ 0 foll >12	2foll>16 ⊕ n foll >12
E2 pg/ml							
>750	S (4)	S (4)	2	1	S (1) (2)		
500-750	S (4)	3	2	1	S (5)	hCG	S (2)
250-500	4	3	2	1		hCG	
150-250	4	3	2	1		hCG	
75-150	3	3	2	1	hCG	hCG	
<75	4	3	3	2 (3) S	S (3)		

FSH
50 -75 IU
x 5 days

Legend	
S STOP	
+100%	% of the starting dose
+50%	
100%	
-50%	
0%	

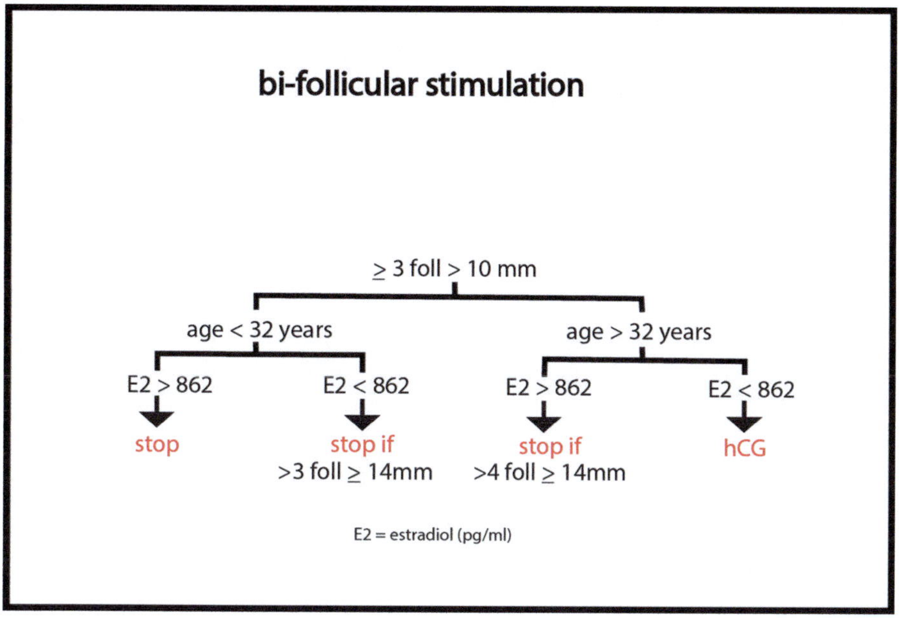

Fig. 10.1 Decision tree for a bifollicular stimulation (From P. Barri [7])

This table illustrates the types of decisions that should be made with various combinations of follicular response (FD mm, *top row*) and plasma estradiol (E2 pg/ml, *left side column*)
Within each box, The *Circle Number* indicates the optimal number of days to continue stimulation, if triggering criteria have not yet been met after 5 days of stimulation. The *Circle Color* indicates the suggested percentage change for FSH dosing in relation to the previous (starting) dose. A *White Circle* with S indicates the cycle should be stopped or abandoned with no further stimulation. Boxes with HCG identify the follicle+estrogen criteria that permit ovulation triggering. Boxes with a number in parentheses refer to 1 of 5 footnotes listed below
When a patient is unable to come in for assessment after the indicated number of days, it remains possible to conduct the monitor one day earlier or later, possibly including a change of the FSH dose
The number of estradiol ranges has been purposely limited in order to simplify the table's construction, and should be considered as approximate when interpretations are made. In particular, when values are close to the indicated upper or lower value of E_2 within a range, the clinical decision should consider options indicated for the adjacent hormone level
Footnotes

1. Triggering with a short-acting GnRH agonist instead of hCG can significantly reduce, but will not eliminate, the risk for OHSS; additional luteal support is then mandatory
2. Triggering with a short-acting GnRH agonist instead of hCG can significantly reduce, but will not eliminate, the risk for multiple pregnancy; additional luteal support is then mandatory
3. Follicular growth that progresses faster than the rise of plasma estradiol levels may be related to an insufficient LH effect; in this case it is better to repeat the stimulation with an FSH preparation that includes LH
4. *Caution*: Risks for OHSS appear and increase when the plasma estradiol level reaches and surpasses 800 pg/ml
5. In this case one may decide either to trigger ovulation, with the expectation that only one ovum will be released, or to abandon the cycle in favor of beginning a new protocol designed to produce two ova

Beware that the couple's attitude may change when a twin pregnancy actually results, even though they may have previously accepted the notion of this "reasonable risk." Whereas the overall pregnancy success rate per cycle increases 30 % when two mature follicles develop, the risk for a multiple pregnancy doubles.

Risk for ovarian hyperstimulation: This risk for this remains low, unless the two mature follicles are accompanied by numerous smaller ones that should be evidenced as plasma estradiol rising above 800 pg/ml. For this reason, the risk is identified with greater confidence.

Criteria for aborting the cycle should be coordinated along with other specific aspects of each patient, e.g., her age, duration of infertility, number of previously unsuccessful stimulation cycles, number and size of secondary follicles in the present cycle, and estradiol levels [6].

Use of *GnRH agonists* is of no value for a bifollicular stimulation. On the other hand, *GnRH antagonists* can be useful along with a plan to delay a single intercourse or an insemination, or to continue FSH stimulation in the presence of a single mature follicle, or if a follicle has developed in an ovary where only the contralateral Fallopian tube is patent.

If a bifollicular cycle is unsuccessful, the same decision-making process applies as is used for monofollicular stimulation protocols. Decisions regarding treatment dosing and duration apply similarly.

10.3 Paucifollicular Stimulation

There are two types of paucifollicular stimulation: unexpected paucifollicular stimulation and intentional paucifollicular stimulation.

10.3.1 Unexpected Paucifollicular Stimulation

A planned mono- or bifollicular stimulation may move out of control. The choice then becomes whether or not to continue with the ovulation trigger according to the prognosis [7].

The prognosis is good for a patient under 32 years of age, or in case of an infertility of less than 3 years' duration: it is possible to work with three follicles, if each is greater than 10 mm diameter, so long as plasma estradiol remains less than 800 pg/ml. The prognosis becomes intermediate for patients between 32 and 38 years of age, or with an infertility of 3–5 years' duration: it may be possible to work with three follicles >14 mm, or with up to six follicles >10 mm, if estradiol continues under 1,000 pg/ml. In a patient over 38 years of age, or with infertility of more than 5 years' duration, the prognosis is poor: it may be possible to work with a third or even a fourth mature follicle, provided the estradiol levels remain under 1,200 pg/ ml.

It is always important to set a purpose and to define safety margins in advance because the greater the number of mature follicles, the higher the pregnancy rate *and also* the multiple pregnancy rate. Belaisch-Allart observed that when the rate of multiple pregnancy dropped from 14.5 to 9.5 % by applying stricter cancelation criteria, the overall pregnancy rate per cycle was also halved, from 21 to 9.5 % [8].

10.3.2 Intentional Paucifollicular Stimulation

Attempts to develop three to five mature follicles can only be justified as part of a plan to compensate with quantity in the face of a poorer quality of oocyte. This typically occurs in patients over 40 years of age. One can design this type of stimulation by combining both components of the bifollicular protocol, namely to start with higher FSH doses (75–125 IU) *and* at an earlier point (CD 3–5). Plasma estradiol should not be allowed to rise much above 800 pg/ml, in order to avoid risk for ovarian hyperstimulation (Table 10.3). A mature follicle number in excess of 2 increases the overall pregnancy rate only slightly, but it significantly increases the risk for a multiple pregnancy [1, 6].

The risks and benefits of paucifollicular stimulation should be discussed in detail with each duly informed couple. Nevertheless, although a poorer oocyte quality rapidly decreases the risks for multiple pregnancy in patients over 38 years of age, this represents just another statistical datum that does not eliminate the potential occurrence of such an unexpected, untoward result. As a matter of fact, such risks would be quite inappropriate for an initial stimulation cycle.

Table 10.3 Managing the standard step-up protocol for a Pauci-follicular stimulation; possible scenarios after administration of 50–75 IU FSH for 5 days (see StimXpert)

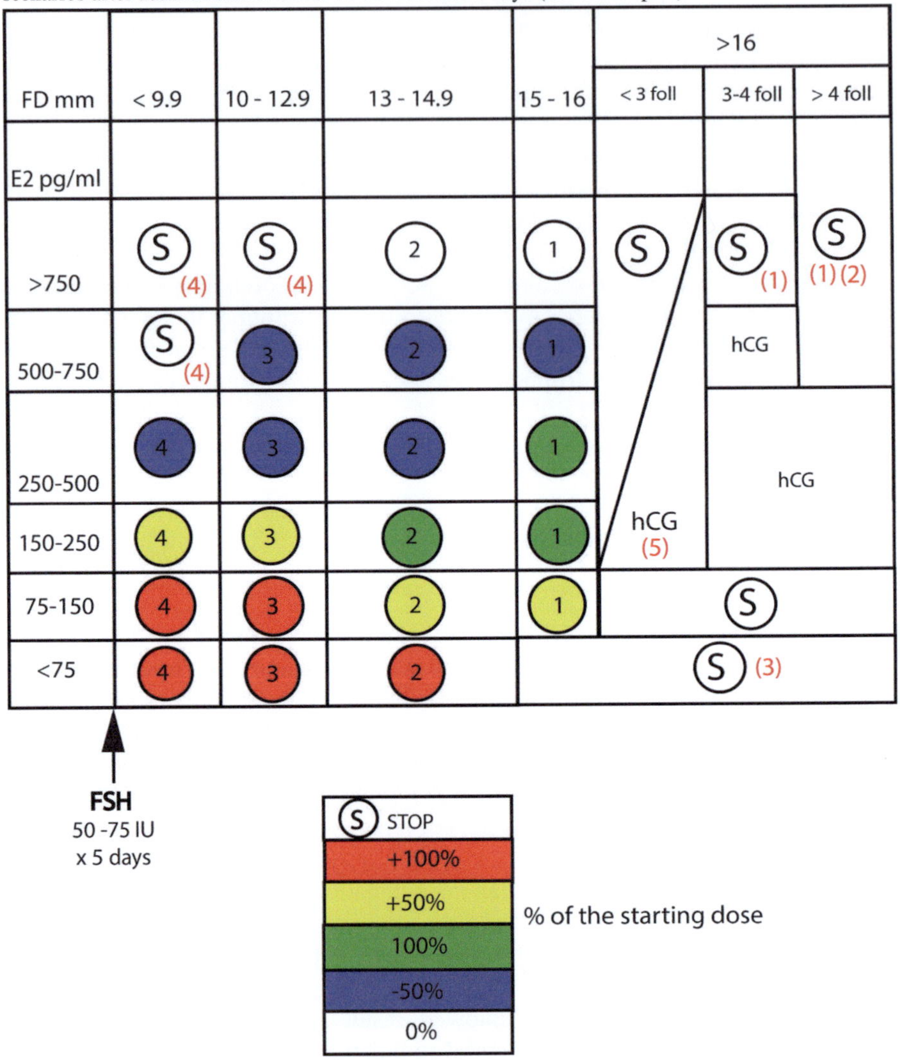

This table illustrates the types of decisions that should be made with various combinations of follicular response (FD mm, *top row*) and plasma estradiol (E_2 pg/ml, *left side column*)
Within each box, The *Circle Number* indicates the optimal number of days to continue stimulation, if triggering criteria have not yet been met after 5 days of stimulation. The *Circle Color* indicates the suggested percentage change for FSH dosing in relation to the previous (starting) dose. A *White Circle* with S indicates the cycle should be stopped or abandoned with no further stimulation. Boxes with HCG identify the follicle+estrogen criteria that permit ovulation triggering. Boxes with a number in parentheses refer to 1 of 5 footnotes listed below
When a patient is unable to come in for assessment after the indicated number of days, it remains possible to conduct the monitor one day earlier or later, possibly including a change of the FSH dose
The number of estradiol ranges has been purposely limited in order to simplify the table's construction, and should be considered as approximate when interpretations are made. In particular, when values are close to the indicated upper or lower value of E_2 within a range, the clinical decision should consider options indicated for the adjacent hormone level
Footnotes

1. Triggering with a short-acting GnRH agonist instead of hCG can significantly reduce, but will not eliminate, the risk for OHSS; additional luteal support is then mandatory
2. Triggering with a short-acting GnRH agonist instead of hCG can significantly reduce, but will not eliminate, the risk for multiple pregnancy; additional luteal support is then mandatory
3. Follicular growth that progresses faster than the rise of plasma estradiol levels may be related to an insufficient LH effect; in this case it is better to repeat the stimulation with an FSH preparation that includes LH
4. *Caution*: Risks for OHSS appear and increase when the plasma estradiol level reaches and surpasses 800 pg/ml
5. In this case one may decide either to trigger ovulation, with the expectation that fewer than three ova will be released, or to abandon the cycle in favor of beginning a new protocol designed to produce three or more ova

References

1. Loumaye E (1995) A phase III, open, randomized multicenter study to compare the safety and efficacy of recombinant human follicle-stimulating hormone (Gonal F) administered subcutaneously with that of urinary human follicle stimulating hormone (Metrodin) given intramuscularly, to induce ovulation in WHO group II anovulatory infertile women. ARES SERONO, Internal Report
2. Dickey RP, Taylor SN, Lu PY et al (2001) Relationship of follicle numbers and estradiol levels to multiple implantation in 3608 intrauterine insemination cycles. Fertil Steril 75:69–78
3. Merviel P, Cedrin-Durnerin I, Belaisch-Allart J et al (2009) Vers la grossesse monofoetale en AMP. Gynecol Obstet Fertil Hors-serie no 1:1–11
4. Antoine JM, Audebert A, Avril C et al (2004) Traitement de la stérilité et grossesses multiple en France: analyses et recommendations. Gynecol Obstet Fertil 32:670–683
5. Cedrin Durnerin I, Massin N, Galey-Fontaine J et al (2006) Timing of FSH administration for ovarian stimulation in normo-ovulatory women: comparison of an early or a mid-follicular phase initiation of a short-term treatment. Hum Reprod 21:2941–2947
6. Belaisch Allart J (2009) Peut-on prévenir les grossesses multiples hors FIV? Gynecol Obstet Fertil 37:6–8
7. Tur R, Barri PN, Coroleu B et al (2005) Use of a prediction model for high-order multiple implantation after ovarian stimulation with gonadotropins. Fertil Steril 83:116–121
8. Belaisch Allart J, Mayenga JM, Grefenstette I et al (2007) Insémination intra-utérine: pourquoi continuer à stimuler l'ovulation? Gynecol Obstet Fertil 35:871–876

11 Stimulation in the Anovulatory Patient

In contrast to the patient who already ovulates spontaneously, the anovulatory patient lacks the benefit of having a cyclic pattern of endogenous gonadotropin secretion. This situation can include a number of aspects that lead to a variety of treatment strategies.

11.1 Characterizing the Anovulation

11.1.1 Clinical Symptoms

Presenting symptoms are typically characterized as menstrual cycle disorders, either as: (1) a permanent amenorrhea, because ovulation is absent, or (2) a spaniomenorrhea, or amenorrhea interspersed with sporadic menstrual bleeding associated with ovulation, or amenorrhea that is secondary to estradiol fluctuations that lead to some endometrial shedding without ovulation having occurred. These bleedings are seldom sufficient and regular enough to mimic normal menstrual cycling.

11.1.2 Etiology

The origin of ovulatory failure is rooted in pituitary FSH secretion:

- Hypogonadotropic anovulation, of hypothalamic-pituitary origin, due to the absence or quasi-absence of FSH and LH secretion (World Health Organization Type I, WHO I)
- Normogonadotropic anovulation, caused either by a qualitative disorder of gonadotropin secretion (WHO IIa) or secondary to an abnormal intra-ovarian folliculogenesis (WHO IIb)
- Hypergonadotropic anovulation corresponding to a vanishing ovarian reserve (WHO III)

J.-C. Emperaire, *Ovulation Stimulation with Gonadotropins*,
DOI 10.1007/978-3-319-18654-2_11

A preliminary etiologic evaluation of the patient should distinguish between these three different types of anovulation, and each will point the way to a therapeutic strategy. The patient workup should encompass at least:

An ultrasound evaluation made between the third and the fifth days of a menstrual bleeding, whether spontaneous or provoked by withdrawal from oral progestins, to clarify the ovarian status and also to conduct an antral follicle count that will distinguish normofollicular from multifollicular ovaries (>25) and paucifollicular (<7) ovaries.

A hormonal evaluation conducted on the same day:

- Dynamic response of FSH and LH, after an injection of 25 μg gonadorelin (*Relfact*®). Serum FSH should raise 100–150 % and LH by 150–200 %, at 60 min post-injection.
- Measures of estradiol, prolactin, TSH, and several androgens: testosterone, Δ^4-androstenedione, dehydroepiandrosterone (DHEA), and DHEA sulfate, and perhaps 17α-hydroxy-progesterone, depending upon the clinical situation. AMH level will usually correlate with AFC.

Because induction of ovulation in a patient whose infertility results from a simple failure to ovulate (pure anovulation) should give her the best chances for a successful pregnancy according to her age, the goal of this procedure must be monofollicular, except in an unusual circumstance.

11.2 Hypogonadotropic Anovulation (Who Type I)

Type I anovulation is characterized by the absence of secretion of both gonadotropins FSH and LH. Because the ovaries are unstimulated they remain at rest, and do not secrete steroids. Likewise, results from a progestin withdrawal test will be negative: due to absence of estrogenic stimulation of the uterine mucosa, a ten-day treatment with oral progestin has no effect (i.e., no withdrawal bleeding).

Anovulation may be considered as primary, where menses have never spontaneously occurred (e.g., with genetic abnormalities such as Kallmann De Morsier Syndrome). It can also be "primary-secondary," where menses did spontaneously begin but then stopped after a few cycles. A secondary anovulation may occur in a woman who apparently ovulated and menstruated normally for some time, but stopped after, for example, discontinuation of oral contraceptives, treatment for a pituitary tumor, or as a component of anorexia nervosa. Often the origin of anovulation remains idiopathic.

11.2.1 Evaluation

Ultrasound examination of these patients typically reveals resting, normofollicular ovaries and a thin quasi-virtual uterine mucosa. Serum FSH and LH are typically very low or undetectable, and a GnRH stimulation test should identify the level of the central disorder. This test distinguishes between anovulation of hypothalamic origin, with FSH-LH secretion appearing under GnRH stimulation, versus a pituitary origin that shows absent gonadotropin response to GnRH. A cranial MRI is mandatory when an organic lesion cannot be ruled out.

Estradiol levels are typically very low, and other related hormone levels will be low to normal. The AMH level is typically normal, but paradoxically may be low in the presence of a normal follicular reserve [1]. A prolactin assay is important to rule out a class of hyperprolactinemic conditions that lead to hypogonadotropic anovulation. Hyperprolactinemia should be treated with dopamine agonists when it is not secondary to an identifiable pituitary tumor, or persists after surgery, and ovarian stimulation by gonadotropins should be undertaken only when the anovulation remains despite prolonged normalization of prolactin levels.

The first line treatment of hypogonadotropic anovulation is the GnRH pump. Pulses of 10–20 μg gonadorelin acetate (*Lutrelef®*) every 90 min should restore normal function of the hypothalamic-pituitary-ovarian axis, without risk of ovarian hyperstimulation, and with low risk for multiple pregnancy. Resorting to direct gonadotropin stimulation should be considered only in cases of known pituitary lesions, in noncompliant patients despite availability of the latest-generation remote-controlled pumps, or in the absence of detectable ovarian response after variations of a suitable GnRH dose and administration frequency.

11.2.2 Treatment Following GnRH

Although the stimulation process in hypogonadotropic patients is fairly straightforward, the challenge remains to find the FSH threshold, and then to lead the selected follicle to full maturity by continuing with gonadotropin administration.

The Gonadotropin: In this situation, stimulation with FSH and LH together becomes necessary because the condition is characterized by the endogenous absence of both hormones. Administration of FSH alone may promote some degree of follicular development in these patients, but the necessary LH-directed estrogen secretion will be insufficient or not present. In addition, cervical mucus and endometrial growth both require adequate estrogen levels. Triggering ovulation of these apparently mature follicles is not likely to result in nidation and pregnancy.

Three mixed gonadotropin preparations are available:

- HMG, with a fixed FSH/LH ratio of one to one
- *Pergoveris®*, having a fixed 2 to 1 FSH/LH ratio that is particularly well suited for this indication. However, the product is available only in vials of 150 IU, which is rather inconvenient because this dose is higher than the FSH threshold of many patients and could result in some product wastage.
- Concomitant administration of FSH and rLH (*Luveris®*). This involves two daily sc injections, but it offers the possibility of adjusting the FSH/LH ratio as needed. A dose of 75 IU rLH seems sufficient to allow for harmonious follicular development in most patients. Higher LH doses are unlikely to disturb the follicular maturation in a hypogonadotropic milieu, so long as the administered FSH/LH ratio does not fall below 1.

Administration Protocol: The step-up low-dose protocol seems in theory to be the best suited for these patients. However, there is a risk for continuing several weeks of one or two daily sc injections at insufficient doses before finding the FSH threshold, although the risk for a multifollicular response is rather low in this situation. For this reason one may initiate with a standard step-up protocol and an initial 7-day stimulation period. This should provoke a good monofollicular response and ovulation in most patients. If this does not succeed initially, the experience still provides a good estimate of ovarian sensitivity to FSH when designing the next cycle that may be shifted to a second line low-dose protocol.

As with all stimulation protocols, the starting dose should be chosen with consideration of the patient's age and BMI: 50 IU in patients under 35 years of age with a normal or low BMI, 75 IU in other cases.

In the standard step-up protocol, stimulation is conducted according to the same principles as the monofollicular stimulation of a spontaneously ovulating patient, but with an initial 7-day treatment period.

If the low-dose step up protocol is used (Table 11.1), initiate treatment between CD2 and CD5, and with a 50–75 IU dose for 7 days. If there is no detectable ovarian response, increase the daily posology by 50 % of the initial dose for another 7 days, and so on, until a dominant follicle appears with a corresponding rise in plasma estradiol. Maintain this same dose until the moment ovulation is triggered. In case of a successful first ovulation but unsuccessful pregnancy, start the next trial with a gonadotropin dose one step *lower* than the observed FSH threshold.

This table illustrates the types of decisions that should be made with various combinations of follicular response (FD mm, *top row*) and plasma estradiol (E_2 pg/ml, *left side column*)

Within each box, The *Circle Number* indicates the optimal number of days to continue stimulation, if triggering criteria have not yet been met after 5 days of stimulation. The *Circle Color* indicates the suggested percentage change for FSH dosing in relation to the previous (starting) dose. A *White Circle* with S indicates the cycle should be stopped or abandoned with no further stimulation. Boxes with HCG identify the follicle + estrogen criteria that permit ovulation triggering. Boxes with a number in parentheses refer to 1 of 4 footnotes listed below

When a patient is unable to come in for assessment after the indicated number of days, it remains possible to conduct the monitor 1 day earlier or later, possibly including a change of the FSH dose

The number of estradiol ranges has been purposely limited in order to simplify the table's construction, and should be considered as approximate when interpreted are made. In particular, when values are close to the indicated upper or lower value of E_2 within a range, the clinical decision should consider options indicated for the adjacent hormone level

Footnotes

1. Triggering with a short-acting GnRH agonist instead of hCG can significantly reduce, but will not eliminate, the risk for OHSS; additional luteal support is then mandatory
2. Triggering with a short-acting GnRH agonist instead of hCG can significantly reduce, but will not eliminate, the risk for multiple pregnancy; additional luteal support is then mandatory
3. Follicular growth that progresses faster than the rise of plasma estradiol levels may be related to an insufficient LH effect; in this case it is better to repeat the stimulation with an FSH preparation that includes LH
4. *Caution*: Risks for OHSS increase to the degree that plasma estradiol surpasses 800 pg/ml

Tiggering Criteria: As with all monofollicular stimulation cycles, the goal is to develop a single follicle >15 mm diameter, without any secondary follicles >12 mm, and with an estradiol level <500 pg/ml. A true hypogonadotropic hypogonadism is the only example of a classical stimulation where a luteal support is sometimes needed. In many cases but not all, the continuing action of hCG administered to

Table 11.1 Managing the low-dose step-up protocol; possible scenarios after administration of 50–75 IU FSH for 7 days (see StimXpert)

FD mm	< 9.9	10 - 12.9	13 - 14.9	15 - 16	>16 1 foll + 0 fol >12	>16 1 foll +n foll >12
E2 pg/ml						
>500	S (4)	3	2	1	S (1) / hCG	S (1) (2)
250 - 500	4	3	2	1	hCG	
150 - 250	4	3	2	1	hCG	
75-150	4	3	2	1	hCG	hCG
<75	7 (5)	4	3	2	S (3)	

FSH
50 -75 IU
x 7 days

Legend	
S STOP	
+100%	% of the starting dose
+50%	
100%	
-50%	
0%	

trigger ovulation provides adequate support for the luteal gland in the absence of pulsatile post-ovulatory LH secretion. It is therefore prudent to monitor post-ovulatory progesterone levels and the luteal phase length during the initial stimulation cycle. When luteal inadequacy is detected, support must be provided either with a progesterone preparation, starting not less than three days after hCG, or with three additional administrations of 750–1,500 IU hCG, at 3 day intervals.

Treatment Duration: In the absence of other hypofertility factors within the couple, the chances for a successful pregnancy in this situation are similar to that of ovulatory couples, through 6–8 stimulation cycles. In case of failure after this, a protocol leading to bifollicular stimulation may be proposed to younger patients for an additional 2–3 cycles before turning to assisted conception. To be sure, this overall strategy and the reasons supporting it should be clearly explained to the couple and accepted by both partners, who often tend to grow impatient after a few ovulatory trials are completed without conception.

11.2.3 Conclusion

Monofollicular stimulation in the hypogonadotropic patient must combine LH with FSH and be administered with a standard or a low-dose step-up protocol. Chances for pregnancy are certainly among the best in all infertility situations, thus a certain amount of support for perseverance is mandatory to avoid the more burdensome process of unwarranted assisted conception.

11.3 Normogonadotropic Anovulation

In these more typical situations, a significant capacity for gonadotropin secretion is present, but it remains nevertheless unable to stimulate sufficient follicular development. Often the source of the disorder lies in the CNS, through perturbations of GnRH pulsatility or of hypothalamic-pituitary-ovarian feedback mechanisms. One of the following situations may be identified:

- Patients with a life style that includes intense physical activity.
- Patients who have chosen diet modification in order to lose weight.
- Patients with pseudo- (or macro-) prolactinemia where measured excessive levels of serum prolactin are actually biologically inactive congregated molecules ("big" and "big-big" prolactin). In these cases, ovulation is not restored after treatment by dopamine agonists.
- Patients treated with psychotropic or neuroleptic drugs that act as dopamine antagonists to disinhibit prolactin secretion.

In most patients, however, the precise origin of inadequate gonadotropin secretion will remain unknown, even when a psychological/behavioral disorder is evoked. In other instances, an ovarian origin can be suspected in the form of a defective folliculogenesis and an accumulation of antral follicles that fail to mature.

These patients typically share two characteristics: (1) A positive response in the oral progestin test because basal gonadotropin secretion has stimulated some follicular estrogenic production that promotes endometrial development capable of responding to progestin administration. (2) A first line treatment of choice by clomiphene citrate (*Clomid*®, *Pergotime*®) – this drug acts as an antagonist at the estrogen receptor level, and raises endogenous gonadotropin secretion by relieving the estrogen-mediated negative feedback at the hypothalamo-pituitary level. In these circumstances, gonadotropin administration should be considered only when clomiphene stimulation fails, either because of failure to ovulate or failure to conceive after ovulation is restored.

In ovulatory failure, a starting dose of clomiphene, 50 mg daily for 5 days, may be progressively increased up to 150 mg when there is no ovarian response. A stepwise increment may be instituted as soon as consecutive cycles in order to benefit from the remaining action of clomiphene, whose half-life can range from 10 days to more than one month, depending upon the isomer considered.

In pregnancy failures, detecting ovulation through monitoring a rise of basal body temperature may be insufficient. An ultrasound examination should be conducted to assess follicular development and rupture, and to indicate when necessary the moment for hCG administration. Consecutive ovulatory cycles without achieving a pregnancy can usually attributed to a subtle anti-estrogenic effect of clomiphene on the endometrium and/or the cervical mucus. In fact the cumulative curve of pregnancy success in patients who ovulate on clomiphene is very close to that of normally ovulating women through 6–9 treatment cycles. Thus clomiphene treatment should be continued for 6 cycles, but not more because of possible risk for long term untoward effects.

Even when ovulation is restored, the estrogen antagonist-related side effects, such as hot flashes or visual disorders, can appear with intensity proportional to the clomiphene dose.

Letrozole, an aromatase inhibitor used principally in patients with breast cancer, can also stimulate ovulation by depletion of endogenous estrogen synthesis, thus increasing gonadotropin secretion. Its potential advantages over clomiphene are the absence of peripheral anti-estrogenic effects, and also a greater success with pregnancy and live birth rates in PCOS patients [2]. However, the drug is not yet authorized for this indication, principally because the potential consequences in offspring are still unknown. There are, however, some reassuring preliminary data [3].

In a situation where gonadotropin stimulation becomes necessary, ovarian appearance at ultrasound should remain the essential assessment for deciding stimulation strategies, and more so than the patient's history, clinical signs and symptoms or the hormonal assays.

11.3.1 Stimulation in Presence of Normofollicular Ovaries

Ultrasound evaluation of patients with hypogonadotropic anovulation and normofollicular ovaries typically show a normal ovarian volume and a total count of 24 or fewer detectable follicles in the two ovaries. Hormone testing reveals low to normal basal gonadotropin levels, a normal FSH-LH response to the GnRH test, and normal levels of prolactin, AMH, TSH and androgens. Despite having some basal secretion of FSH and LH, these patients fall somewhere between hypogonadotropic hypogonadism and normally ovulating women. Plans for ovarian stimulation should be designed along the lines of treating both situations.

Clomiphene citrate is well suited for these patients, who already have some endogenous estrogen expression. If clomiphene is unsuccessful, the GnRH pump may be able to restore normal gonadotropin dynamics, although efficacy may actually be lower than in cases of complete gonadotropin absence. Administration of gonadotropins thus becomes the last resort when both clomiphene and GnRH have failed. Any of the FSH gonadotropin preparations are equally useful, because the patient has sufficient endogenous LH secretion.

The first-line protocol for gonadotropin stimulation should be the standard step-up protocol, and it should achieve success with relatively few injections and monitoring steps. In case of failure, depending upon the observed ovarian response, one may repeat the same protocol with a different starting dose or move to a step-up low-dose protocol (Table 11.1). Triggering criteria are those used for monofollicular cycles: a single follicle with a mean diameter >15 mm and without other follicles >12 mm diameter, together with an estradiol level between 150 and 350 pg/ml. Luteal support is not necessary, unless a short luteal phase defect has been noted, and/or if serum progesterone persists below 10 ng/ml. It should be possible to repeat gonadotropin stimulations for at least 6 cycles in young patients, so long as the procedure provokes a satisfactory ovulation during each cycle.

11.3.2 Stimulation in Presence of Multifollicular Ovaries

The multifollicular situation (AFC >24) encompasses many of the principal difficulties of attempting ovarian stimulation. Because of numerous risks for a rapid excessive response, more sophisticated stimulation protocols have been designed to achieve success with this situation. The syndrome is already characterized by disturbed folliculogenesis and an overabundance of follicles capable of selection, with anti-Mullerian hormone and androgens playing a significant role. While the true origin of the disorder remains essentially obscure, two distinct types can be revealed at ultrasound:

"Simple" multifollicular ovaries, which are only slightly enlarged, containing numerous follicles of various sizes distributed within the whole ovarian parenchyma, and with a normal stroma (Fig. 11.1).

Micropolycystic ovaries, usually enlarged, with large numbers of small to very small follicles tightly packed under the ovarian albuginea, and with a compact, echogenic stroma (Fig. 11.2).

An intermediate or combined appearance of both is also possible, and it may be difficult to define clearly the presence of a compact stroma. This explains the tribulations endured by those attempting to establish specific ultrasound criteria for the

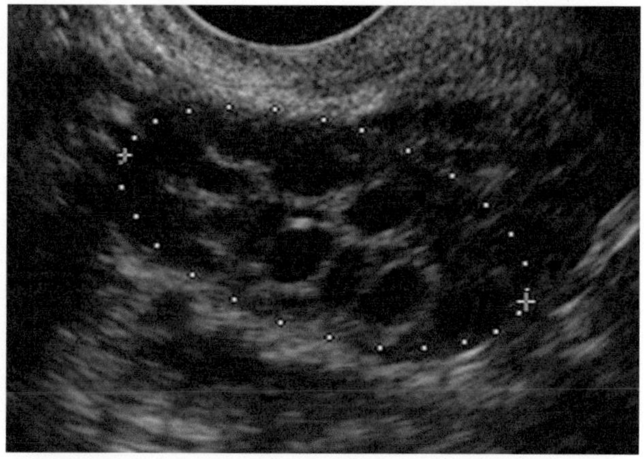

Fig. 11.1 Ultrasound appearance of multifollicular ovaries: numerous follicles of different sizes are located throughout the ovarian parenchyma (Photo courtesy of B. Broussin)

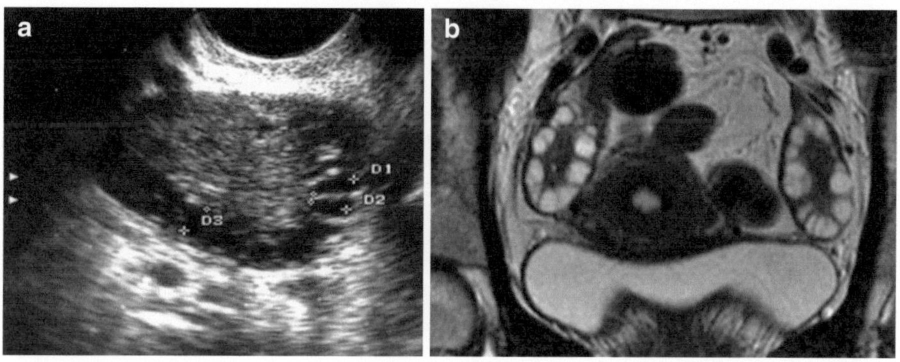

Fig. 11.2 Micropolycystic ovaries: numerous small follicles are compressed under the tunica albuginea at the periphery of the ovary. Appearance at ultrasound (**a**) and MRI (**b**). (Images Courtesy P. Billet)

various diagnoses. Initially absent from the First NIH Consensus Conference Proceedings (1990), the ultrasound criteria have become more refined as a result of the ESHRE Consensus Conference (Rotterdam 2003) [4]. At present, multifollicular syndromes comprise the classic polycystic ovarian syndrome (PCOS), with its spectrum of clinical, biological, and metabolic criteria, while other multifollicular ovarian presentations constitute an exclusion diagnosis. On the practical level, however, the appearance at ultrasound of a total count of more than 25 follicles in both ovaries, together with a high AMH level, should alert a clinician for a potentially excessive response to stimulation, regardless of the clinical and biological context.

PCOS was first described by Stein and Leventhal as polycystic ovaries in the presence of three principal features: anovulation, obesity and hyperandrogenism,

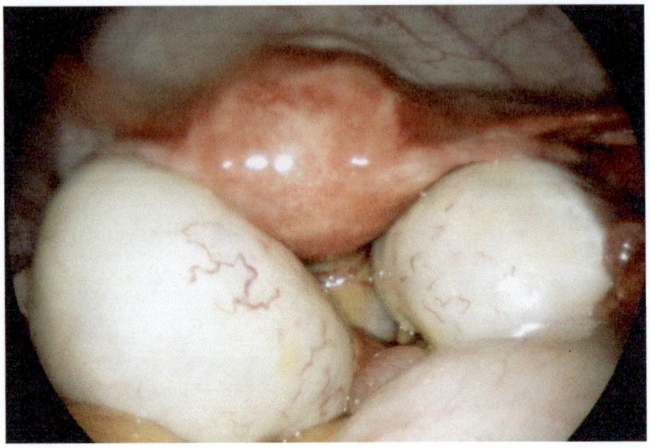

Fig. 11.3 The "billiard balls" appearance of polycystic ovaries at laparoscopy (Photo courtesy of R.B. Greenblatt)

whether or not clinically apparent [5]. In the absence of ultrasound imaging at that time, diagnosis was usually confirmed by laparoscopy that revealed markedly enlarged white nacreous ovaries, giving the impression, along with the uterus, of the three billiard balls (Fig. 11.3). Cuneiform resection of the ovaries in order to restore ovulation showed numerous small follicles packed under a very thick tunica albuginea.

Currently, to be considered as having PCOS, the patient should present with two of the three following features (Rotterdam consensus criteria [6]:

- Anovulation or oligo-ovulation
- Clinical and/or biological hyperandrogenism
- More than a dozen follicles per ovary

The third of these criteria, while of utmost importance, is somewhat imprecise, because measures are often operator and/or equipment-dependent. Latest-generation 3-dimensional equipment can detect ever smaller follicles of less than 2 mm. A true count of 20 or even 25 follicles per ovary seems more likely the current norm for PCOS [6].

It remains possible that the diagnosis of PCOS, named essentially because of the ovarian appearance, may paradoxically be established without sonographic criteria. An apparent contradiction occurs because normofollicular ovaries may respond to ovarian stimulation like typical polycystic ovaries, yet other patients diagnosed by ultrasound with typical PCOS may occasionally respond to stimulation as one with normofollicular ovaries.

Additional clinical features of PCOS may include hyperandrogenism characterized by acne, hypertrichosis, or true hirsutism, and obesity or an elevated BMI, either as a female type or the androgynous type associated with hyperandrogenism.

Endocrine testing may show:

- Increased plasma LH with an inversion of the FSH/LH ratio, and an excessive LH response to the dynamic GnRH test.
- Elevated testosterone and Δ^4-androstenedione – an assay of 17-hydroxy-progesterone is recommended to rule out an incomplete blockage of adrenal steroid synthesis.
- An AMH level over 5 ng/ml is also very suggestive; measures of this hormone are indeed becoming a fourth important criterion for establishing the PCOS diagnosis [7]. Elevated AMH might indeed is one of the main causes of PCOS, instead of a simple indicator of the condition [8].
- Hyperinsulinism that enhances the LH effect on androgen secretion along with a possible dyslipidemia and/or hypertension. PCOS is often characterized as a variant form of metabolic syndrome.

11.3.3 Treatment of PCOS

Several options may be considered, in a progressive strategy.

The GnRH pump, which may be chosen initially or after a failure with clomiphene. However, results for PCOS have not been promising to date, and it should be relegated to isolated cases.

Clomiphene citrate remains the first line therapy, after or along with metformin therapy in cases of obesity with hyperinsulinism. Letrozole seems to work as well, but its use for this indication remains a matter of debate.

Ovarian drilling, which is simply an update of the concept underlying the former wedge resection approach. This is a strategy whose mode of action has never been fully explained, yet it restores spontaneous ovulatory cycles to some 80 % of patients. With laparoscopic guidance, several small punctures are inserted into each ovary. In some series, pregnancy rates of 50 % have been observed within the first year [9]. Nonetheless, anovulation eventually returns, and new trials with clomiphene citrate, to which the ovary may have been sensitized by the drilling process, are worth considering. If this fails, a second drilling may be proposed to the patient, although with a caution of diminished expectations.

The principal value of ovarian drilling is that it can restore spontaneous ovulations and chances for a normal pregnancy without increasing the risk of ovarian hyperstimulation. Another useful and valuable outcome is that the risk of multiple pregnancy is comparable to that of spontaneously ovulating woman. On the other hand, the laparoscopy itself is a significant drawback because it is an invasive exploration of the abdomen with numerous attendant hazards from anesthesia. Modern technology has now greatly reduced complications from pelvic adhesions.

Should clomiphene trials fail, ovarian drilling may be advisable in several circumstances:

- During a laparoscopy for another purpose, e.g. to follow up on an abnormal hysterosalpingogram or when pelvic endometriosis is suspected.
- In PCOD patients who may not be sufficiently compliant for a protocol of repeated gonadotropin injections and monitoring steps.
- In patients who have the best chance for success with this procedure: BMI <35, infertility duration less than 3 years, a negligible hyperandrogenism, and serum LH <10 mIU/ml [10].
- Drilling may also be considered for a patient who continually develops multifollicular responses with gonadotropins, no matter how cautious the injection protocol.

Gonadotropin treatment remains the most difficult aspect of stimulation in PCOS patients because, by definition, their ovaries already contain a large pool of preantral follicles with a very close sensitivity to FSH. The margin of safety, between the threshold of FSH and the level causing an excessive response is narrow; several follicles can easily be recruited as soon as the FSH threshold is reached, or at only slightly higher doses. It is prudent to expect an excessive response and to proceed very cautiously with a progressive stimulation, even if surprisingly moderate responses should appear as well.

Choice of gonadotropin: In theory, purified FSH preparations would seem to be best suited for these patients, who already have elevated endogenous LH. Indeed, highly purified u-FSH preparations were originally designed for stimulating ovulation in the PCOS patient. Furthermore, one must also be concerned with an LH ceiling, above which an excess is deleterious to the chances for a normally developing pregnancy [11]. Nevertheless, use of regular HMG yields in fact the same rate as purified FSH for successful pregnancy as well as for miscarriage. All FSH preparations are equally effective for PCOS, as if the added LH were not able to breach the hypothetical LH ceiling.

Administration protocol: The starting dose should be 50–75 IU, depending upon the patient's age and BMI, but a standard step-up approach is certainly not well suited for this indication. On the other hand, because many criteria for estimating ovarian response are imprecise, a fear of excessive response may lead paradoxically to insufficient stimulation over prolonged periods. A step-up low-dose protocol remains the best first line approach for PCOS. If a plurifollicular response continues after reaching the FSH threshold, other protocols are then possible:

- The step-up chronic low-dose protocol, designed to maintain the starting dose for 7 additional days when the first 7 days failed to elicit an ovarian response. Dose increments continue for 7-day intervals (Table 11.2). If excessive follicular recruitment should appear, one can reduce the starting dose or the increment percentage from one stage to the next (e.g., a step-up chronic ultra-low dose protocol).

- If inadequate results persist, the next approach would be a sequential protocol, i.e., *reducing* the FSH dose once follicle dominance is reached, thereby to diminish the risk of recruiting secondary follicles. This approach can be tricky to manage: reducing the dose too late will end in another failure, whereas reducing it too early will simply result in a general follicular atresia (Table 11.3).
- If all of the progressive protocols fail, it would be possible to attempt a step-down protocol, which works along inverse principles. A higher initial dose (100–150 IU) results in a deliberate plurifollicular recruitment, and the secondary reduction in FSH leads to development of only the most sensitive follicle. Some clinicians prefer this protocol as a first line stimulation, but substantial experience is necessary to choose with confidence the very moment when FSH dosing should be reduced (Table 11.4).
- In patients without PCOS, estradiol production reaches a maximum at 6 h after a single FSH injection, and is maintained at this level for at least 24 h. In PCOS patients, the maximum estradiol production begins to decline sooner, by 12 h after FSH, and at 24 h post-FSH estradiol production is only 40 % of the maximal level. Unfortunately, splitting the FSH dose for a twice-daily administration does not appear to improve the clinical results [12].

Triggering criteria for a monofollicular stimulation are unchanged: one seeks a single follicle >15 mm diameter in the absence of other follicles >12 mm. Recall that PCOS ovaries contain numerous small follicles that all contribute to the total estrogen secretion, which still needs to remain below 800 pg/ml in order to obviate risk for ovarian hyperstimulation. If risk does appear, merely skipping the hCG trigger may not be sufficient to avoid multiple pregnancy for these at-risk patients. Contraceptive measures are strongly recommended for a length of time [13].

If the step-up protocols fail:

- When a pregnancy does not follow a cycle that did result in an adequate ovulation, one may use the same FSH doses in additional cycles.
- If different step-up protocols all fail with a persistent plurifollicular response, even in the face of slower step-up chronic low-dose protocol, it may still be possible to repeat cycles at diminished starting doses and/or with smaller dose increases for subsequent stages.
- An insufficient response, on the other hand, may require shifting to a less progressive protocol, or to an increased starting dose and/or to a larger dose increment between each stage.

If the step-down or sequential protocols fail, the cycle may be abandoned for one of two reasons, both tied to the timing of the dose reduction. If the response is plurifollicular, the reduction of FSH dose was either insufficient or too late. On the other hand, follicular atresia usually follows an FSH dose reduction that was too early or too great. Noting the details of inadequate responses will guide management of the next stimulation cycle. If difficulties continue despite corrections of timing and dosing, it is better to change the protocol altogether.

Table 11.2 Managing the chronic low-dose step-up protocol: possible scenarios after administration of 50–75 IU FSH for 7 days (see StimXpert)

FD mm	< 9.9	10 - 12.9	13 - 14.9	15 - 16	>16 1 foll >16 + 0 foll > 12	>16 1 foll >16 + n foll >12
E2 pg/ml						
>500	S (4)	3	2	1	S (1) / hCG	S (1) (2)
250 - 500	4	3	2	1		
150 - 250	4	3	2	1	hCG	
75-150	4	3	2	1	hCG	hCG
<75	7 / 7 (5)	4	3	2	S (3)	

FSH
50 -75 IU
x 7 days

S STOP
+100%
+50%
100%
-50%
0%

% of the starting dose

Finally, the appearance of polycystic ovaries on ultrasound, with or without other signs of PCOS, should lead one to expect a possible plurifollicular response, and to adjust the administration protocol and FSH dosing appropriately. Even at the cost of a few initial failures, the ability to select from a variety of available protocols should lead to an effective monofollicular ovulatory response in every patient. When the stimulation failures continue for some reason, one should then reconsider the possibility of ovarian drilling, if not previously performed, or alternatively to consider in vitro fertilization as a last resort. Indeed, the excessive ovarian response may be used to some advantage in this situation.

11.3.4 (Apparently) Simple Multifollicular Ovaries

Ovarian reactions may shift between normal and multifollicular responses, due to the variety of beginning forms, transition forms and mixed forms with PCOS. For some authors, these asymptomatic patients, that range from 10 to 30 %, depending

◄

This table illustrates the types of decisions that should be made with various combinations of follicular response (FD mm, *top row*) and plasma estradiol (E_2 pg/ml, *left side column*)
Within each box, The *Circle Number* indicates the optimal number of days to continue stimulation, if triggering criteria have not yet been met after 7 days of stimulation. The *Circle Color* indicates the suggested percentage change for FSH dosing in relation to the previous (starting) dose. A *White Circle* with S indicates the cycle should be stopped or abandoned with no further stimulation. Boxes with HCG identify the follicle + estrogen criteria that permit ovulation triggering. Boxes with a number in parentheses refer to 1 of 4 footnotes listed below
When a patient is unable to come in for assessment after the indicated number of days, it remains possible to conduct the monitor 1 day earlier or later, possibly including a change of the FSH dose
The number of estradiol ranges has been purposely limited in order to simplify the table's construction, and should be considered as approximate when interpreted are made. In particular, when values are close to the indicated upper or lower value of E_2 within a range, the clinical decision should consider options indicated for the adjacent hormone level
Footnotes

1. Triggering with a short-acting GnRH agonist instead of hCG can significantly reduce, but will not eliminate, the risk for OHSS; additional luteal support is then mandatory
2. Triggering with a short-acting GnRH agonist instead of hCG can significantly reduce, but will not eliminate, the risk for multiple pregnancy; additional luteal support is then mandatory
3. Follicular growth that progresses faster than the rise of plasma estradiol levels may be related to an insufficient LH effect; in this case it is better to repeat the stimulation with an FSH preparation that includes LH
4. *Caution*: Risks for OHSS increase to the degree that plasma estradiol surpasses 800 pg/ml

Table 11.3 Managing the sequential step-up/step-down protocol: possible scenarios after administration of 50–75 IU FSH for 7 days (see StimXpert)

FD mm	< 9.9	10 - 12.9	13 - 14.9	15 - 16	>16: 1 foll >16 + 0 foll > 12	>16: 1 foll >16 + n foll >12
E2 pg/ml						
>750	S (4)	S (4)	2	1	S (1)	S (1) (2)
500-750	4	2	3	1	hCG	
250-500	3	2	2	1	hCG	
150-250	4	2	2	1	hCG	
75-150	7 (5)	2	2	1	hCG	
<75	7 (5)	3	2	S (3)		

FSH
50 -75 IU
x 7 days

% of the starting dose
S STOP
+100%
+50%
100%
-50%
0%

upon the discrimination power of the ultrasound equipment, should be considered as moderate or silent forms of PCOS [2]. A standard step-up protocol is best suited to evaluate the patient's response quickly, involving only a few injections with few monitoring controls. Even if it results an initial ovulatory failure, observations of the initial ovarian reaction aids the planning of future cycles.

11.3.5 Paucifollicular Ovaries

A paucifollicular condition is defined as the appearance at ultrasound of a follicular total count equal to or less than six within both ovaries, during the initial stimulation cycle. This is seen more frequently in patients over 38 years of age, or at any age when accompanied by other irregularities of ovarian reserve.

For these situations, classic stimulation protocols are not at all unsuitable. A standard step-up protocol, at the usual or a slightly increased starting dose (e.g., 100–150 IU FSH), will provoke a mono- or paucifollicular response in most cases.

This table illustrates the types of decisions that should be made with various combinations of follicular response (FD mm, *top row*) and plasma estradiol (E_2 pg/ml, *left side column*)
Within each box, The *Circle Number* indicates the optimal number of days to continue stimulation, if triggering criteria have not yet been met after 7 days of stimulation. The *Circle Color* indicates the suggested percentage change for FSH dosing in relation to the previous (starting) dose. A *White Circle* with S indicates the cycle should be stopped or abandoned with no further stimulation. Boxes with HCG identify the follicle+estrogen criteria that permit ovulation triggering. Boxes with a number in parentheses refer to 1 of 4 footnotes listed below
When a patient is unable to come in for assessment after the indicated number of days, it remains possible to conduct the monitor 1 day earlier or later, possibly including a change of the FSH dose
The number of estradiol ranges has been purposely limited in order to simplify the table's construction, and should be considered as approximate when interpreted are made. In particular, when values are close to the indicated upper or lower value of E_2 within a range, the clinical decision should consider options indicated for the adjacent hormone level
Footnotes

1. Triggering with a short-acting GnRH agonist instead of hCG can significantly reduce, but will not eliminate, the risk for OHSS; additional luteal support is then mandatory
2. Triggering with a short-acting GnRH agonist instead of hCG can significantly reduce, but will not eliminate, the risk for multiple pregnancy; additional luteal support is then mandatory
3. Follicular growth that progresses faster than the rise of plasma estradiol levels may be related to an insufficient LH effect; in this case it is better to repeat the stimulation with an FSH preparation that includes LH
4. *Caution*: Risks for OHSS increase to the degree that plasma estradiol surpasses 800 pg/ml

Table 11.4 Managing the step-down protocol: possible scenarios after administration of 150 IU FSH for 5 days (see StimXpert)

FD mm	< 9.9	10 - 12.9	13 - 14.9	15 - 16	>16 1 foll >16 + 0 foll > 12	>16 1 foll >16 + n foll >12
E2 pg/ml						
>750	S (4)	S (4)	1	1	hCG	S (1) (2)
500-750	S (4)	3	2	1	hCG	
250-500	5 (6)	3	2	1	hCG	
150-250	5	3 (6)	2 (6)	1 (6)	hCG	
75-150	5	3 (6)	2 (6)	1 (6)	hCG	
<75	5 (5)	3 (6)	2 (6)	1 (6)	S (3)	

FSH
150 IU
x 5 days

S STOP
+100%
+50%
100%
-25%
-50%
0%

% of the starting dose

Should the ovarian reaction prove to be insufficient, it is acceptable to increase the dose, without fear of an excessive response. In this condition, the problem is less with the ovarian response than with quality of the oocytes themselves, which remains unresponsive to any type of stimulation. Prior to beginning any stimulation it is critically important to decide with the patient about acceptable limits of treatment, and with the understanding that a pleasant surprise always remains possible.

11.4 Hypergonadotropic Anovulations

Hypergonadotropic anovulation is a distinct contraindication for gonadotropin treatment. The combination of continually elevated FSH levels, together with an AMH <0.5 ng/ml, and the appearance of an occasional follicle at ultrasound, are all associated with a premature pre-menopause. High FSH levels are the consequence of diminished feedback due to diminished ovarian responsiveness, and this cannot be relieved by administration of more FSH.

This table illustrates the types of decisions that should be made with various combinations of follicular response (FD mm, *top row*) and plasma estradiol (E_2 pg/ml, *left side column*)
Within each box, The *Circle Number* indicates the optimal number of days to continue stimulation, if triggering criteria have not yet been met after 5 days of stimulation. The *Circle Color* indicates the suggested percentage change for FSH dosing in relation to the previous (starting) dose. A *White Circle* with S indicates the cycle should be stopped or abandoned with no further stimulation. Boxes with HCG identify the follicle+estrogen criteria that permit ovulation triggering. Boxes with a number in parentheses refer to 1 of 5 footnotes listed below
When a patient is unable to come in for assessment after the indicated number of days, it remains possible to conduct the monitor 1 day earlier or later, possibly including a change of the FSH dose
The number of estradiol ranges has been purposely limited in order to simplify the table's construction, and should be considered as approximate when interpreted are made. In particular, when values are close to the indicated upper or lower value of E_2 within a range, the clinical decision should consider options indicated for the adjacent hormone level
Footnotes

1. Triggering with a short-acting GnRH agonist instead of hCG can significantly reduce, but will not eliminate, the risk for OHSS; additional luteal support is then mandatory
2. Triggering with a short-acting GnRH agonist instead of hCG can significantly reduce, but will not eliminate, the risk for multiple pregnancy; additional luteal support is then mandatory
3. Follicular growth that progresses faster than the rise of plasma estradiol levels may be related to an insufficient LH effect; in this case it is better to repeat the stimulation with an FSH preparation that includes LH
4. *Caution*: Risks for OHSS increase to the degree that plasma estradiol surpasses 800 pg/ml
5. The daily dose of FSH should not fall below 75 IU

Many treatment schedules have been proposed in an attempt to manage this most frustrating situation in younger women, often using high doses of administered FSH following a return to normal endogenous FSH levels through treatment with estradiol or a GnRH agonist preparation. However, the proclaimed rates of success do not exceed the number of spontaneous pregnancies that follow a simple estrogen-progestin therapy that is recommended in any case for prevention of osteoporosis. While oocyte donation may be the only realistic option for these patients, two additional points should be emphasized:

- Moderately elevated FSH levels (<15 IU/l) may simply be the result of an FSH receptor mutation, which in this case could justify an attempt with additional gonadotropins. Either a normal ovulation will occur with higher than usual FSH doses over several cycles, because the oocyte quality itself is most likely normal, or no response will occur, and the treatment should then be abandoned.
- The diagnosis of premature menopause should lead to a thorough exploration in search of its origin, particularly if genetic or immunologic aspects could be involved. Although a precise diagnosis will not change the reproductive outcome, some possible etiologies may have other medical consequences.

References

1. Chan C, Liu K (2014) Clinical pregnancy in a woman with idiopathic hypogonadotropic hypogonadism and low AMH: utility of ovarian reserve markers in IHH. J Assist Reprod Genet 31(10):1317–1321
2. Legro RS, Brzyski RG, Diamond MP et al (2014) Letrozole versus clomiphene for infertility in the polycystic ovary syndrome. N Engl J Med 371:119–129
3. Sharma S, Ghosh S, Singh S et al (2014) Congenital malformations among babies born following letrozole or clomiphene for infertility treatment. PLoS One 9(10):e108219
4. The Rotterdam ESHRE/ASRM Sponsored PCOS consensus workshop group (2004) Revised 2003 consensus on diagnostic criteria and long-term health risks related to polycystic ovary syndrome (PCOS). Hum Reprod 19:41–47
5. Stein I, Leventhal M (1935) Amenorrhea associated with bilateral polycystic ovaries. Am J Obstet Gynecol 29:181–185
6. Dewailly D, Gronier H, Poncelet E et al (2011) Diagnosis of Polycystic Ovary Syndrome (PCOS): revisiting the threshold values of follicle count and the serum AMH level for the definition of polycystic ovaries. Hum Reprod 26:3123–3129
7. Lauritsen MP, Pinborg A, Loft A et al (2015) Revised criteria for PCOS in WHO Group II anovulatory infertility–a revival of hypothalamic amenorrhea? Clin Endocrinol (Oxf) 82(4):584–591
8. Homburg R, Crawford G (2014) The role of AMH in anovulation associated with PCOS: a hypothesis. Hum Reprod 29:1117–1121
9. Mayenga JM, Grzegorczyk MV, Belaisch-Allart J (2011) Place actuelle du drilling ovarien dans la prise en charge du syndrome des ovaires polykystiques. Gynecol Obstet Fertil 39:518–520
10. Amer S, Li TC, Ledger WL (2004) Ovulation induction using laparoscopic ovarian drilling in women with polycystic ovarian syndrome: predictors of success. Hum Reprod 19:1719–1724

11. Loumaye E, Engrand P, Shoham Z et al (2003) Clinical evidence for an LH ceiling? Hum Reprod 18:2719–2720
12. Dahan MH, Lathi R (2014) Twice-daily dosing of gonadotropins does not improve embryo quality during in vitro fertilization cycles in women with polycystic ovary syndrome, compared with once-daily dosing: a pilot study. Arch Gynecol Obstet 289:1113–1118
13. Lipitz S, Ben Rafael Z, Bider D et al (1991) Quintuplet pregnancy and third degree ovarian hyperstimulation despite withholding human chorionic gonadotropin. Hum Reprod 6:1478–1479

Multifollicular Stimulation 12

For in vitro fertilization (IVF), the process of ovarian stimulation includes some unique yet essential contrasts to the methods for classic mono- or pauci-follicular stimulations.

First and foremost, this process is a multifollicular stimulation. Even if only a single embryo is to be transferred, IVF typically seeks to collect several oocytes in order to provide an optimal choice of embryo for transfer, as well as to enable frozen preservation of supernumerary high quality embryos for possible transfer at a later time.

Therefore, this procedure should be considered as a *deliberate* ovarian hyperstimulation. It should be fully expected, if hCG is administered, that the excessive quantity of follicles of all sizes, developing in both ovaries, together with the resulting estrogen secretion, will expose the patient to well-identified risks for an ovarian hyperstimulation syndrome. A safe process is made possible solely because oocyte harvesting evacuates the follicular contents and diminishes the chain of events leading to an OHSS. This procedure is in effect a controlled expansion of the safety limits.

Ovarian stimulation is only one of several aspects necessary for a successful outcome from IVF. Chances for pregnancy are very dependent on high standards and quality in the embryology laboratory. While a high-grade laboratory can compensate to an extent for suboptimal oocyte quality, the reverse is not true. The best-run stimulation protocol will be of little value in the face of inadequate embyrology procedures. For this reason, stimulation quality in IVF correlates less well with successful pregnancy rates than do most classic stimulations.

This multifollicular stimulation, or rather, this controlled ovarian hyperstimulation (COH) is realized by manipulating two of the usual rules that control follicular recruitment and development (Fig. 12.1): (1) Administration of supra-physiologic gonadotropin doses as soon as the first days of the cycle, which quickly exceeds the FSH threshold and recruits more elements of the follicular pool. (2) Continuation of these high doses throughout the stimulation period to prevent closure of the FSH window, thereby sustaining a complete development and maturation of most of the recruited follicles.

J.-C. Emperaire, *Ovulation Stimulation with Gonadotropins*,
DOI 10.1007/978-3-319-18654-2_12

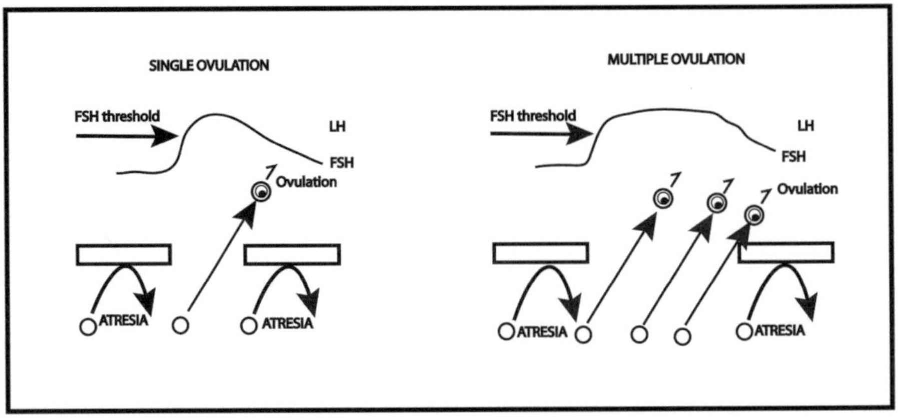

Fig. 12.1 Comparison of the classical and multifollicular ovarian stimulation

12.1 Evolution of Ovarian Stimulation Protocols for IVF

Having abandoned the use of clomiphene for ovarian stimulation, Edwards and Steptoe turned next to a low dose gonadotropin stimulation, but left this approach as well because they felt that it led to implantation failures. Their first successful IVF pregnancy in 1978 was actually the result of a spontaneous ovulation that simply involved monitoring the urinary peak of LH to identify the proper moment for oocyte harvest [1]. Once the feasibility of IVF was demonstrated, additional teams decided to stimulate ovulation with the goal of producing more oocytes and more suitable embryos for transfer.

12.1.1 Stimulation Protocols

Initially, two distinct stimulation protocols came into use [2]:

The Clomiphene-HMG protocol, more commonly used in Europe: Oral clomiphene citrate, 100 mg daily, was administered for 5 days, starting on CD2, followed by injections of 225 IU HMG on CD 3, 5, and 7, and with the initial first monitoring assessment conducted on CD 9.

The HMG-Only protocol, more commonly adopted in the USA: This model was notably developed and used by Drs. Georgiana and Howard Jones, and consisted simply of injections with 150–225 IU HMG daily from CD 2 or 3, and initial monitoring controls made on CD 7–8.

In fact, both protocols had a pair of blatant drawbacks: one was that it resulted in the production of asynchronous follicles of many sizes. In addition, untimely LH surges promoted by supra-physiologic estrogen secretion from the numerous follicles led to premature luteinization and/or to an ovulatory process fraught with difficulties in choosing the precise timing for oocyte harvest. As a result many cycles had to be cancelled.

Furthermore, management of these protocols was somewhat challenging. hCG administration should ideally be done at the precise moment when sufficient numbers of follicles are mature, but before a *spontaneous* gonadotropin surge provoked by the most advanced follicle begins to halt the development of intermediary follicles. This difficult task often led to a disappointing oocyte yield or to an overly high rate, some 15 %, of cancelled cycles. Successful pregnancy rates, taking into account all degrees of hCG elevation, were only 15–25 % per transfer, although poor performance of embryology laboratories during this era undoubtedly played a role in overall results. At the present time one should expect rates at least twice as high, now that these protocols are enhanced by GnRH antagonists.

12.1.2 Use of GnRH Agonists

The appearance of GnRH agonists in 1986 revolutionized protocols of ovarian stimulation for IVF purposes because the agonists suppress the potential for LH surges and thereby improve management of the stimulation process. Out of this principle, two new protocol designs appeared at virtually the same moment:

The Short Agonist Protocol, that exploited the initial "flare-up" effect of a short-lived agonist. It quickly fell from favor because its pregnancy rates were only marginally better than those of previous protocols not using GnRH analogs. While the long agonist protocol rates are now clearly superior, the short agonist approach remains as a possible last resort for certain poor responders.

The Long Agonist Protocol, that can be considered as an ovarian stimulation after a preliminary desensitization. This approach has resulted in a clear augmentation of successful pregnancy rates, and has now risen to become the gold standard of ovarian stimulation for IVF purposes.

In contrast to earlier protocols, a more homogeneous follicular cohort results from this long agonist protocol. To be sure, a distinctly greater total gonadotropin dose is necessary to stimulate development and maturation of follicles in a previously desensitized ovary. However, the absence of premature LH surges together with the homogeneous follicle cohort allows selection of more oocytes and leads to higher pregnancy rates. The period for follicle recruitment is also extended. It must also be acknowledged that follicular cohort sizes and plasma estradiol levels are much higher than previously known during stimulation protocols, and this is accompanied by a higher risk for ovarian hyperstimulation.

Because of these enhanced risks for hyperstimulation and also multiple pregnancies following the transfer of several embryos, and also because of modern success with embryo freezing, clinicians are now being urged to consider a single embryo transfer (SET) and to freeze the supernumerary good quality embryos. This reduces the need for multifollicular stimulation cohorts and results in milder ("soft," "friendly") stimulation protocols.

The appearance of GnRH antagonists in 1999 could not have come at a better time to enhance this strategy because daily antagonist administration only prevents premature LH surges. Without the preliminary desensitization, the follicular cohort becomes more heterogeneous and smaller in number than with GnRH agonists. Despite a smaller number of oocytes, pregnancy rates remain comparable to those from agonist use but are made possible within a more moderate stimulation protocol. Moreover, risks for ovarian hyperstimulation are dramatically reduced because ovulation may be triggered when necessary using a short lived GnRH agonist.

Use of GnRH antagonists finally brings in the advantages of earlier multifollicular stimulation protocols that were in use before the appearance of GnRH agonists. Thanks to adequate control of the LH levels, it is once again possible to develop a sufficient number of mature oocytes and realize customary pregnancy success rates, but without the drawbacks of the long agonist protocol. On the other hand, management of antagonist stimulation is somewhat more challenging than with agonist protocols. Deciding on the precise moment to introduce the antagonist, at least in the flexible protocol, becomes crucial.

12.2 The Multifollicular Stimulation Protocol for IVF

At the present time, follicular stimulation for IVF purposes (controlled ovarian hyperstimulation, COH) should use both gonadotropins and a GnRH analogue in tandem to prevent a misplaced ovulation or a premature luteinization.

12.2.1 Preliminary Steps

Evaluations and preparations for stimulation are not different from those for a classic stimulation; numerous factors such as tobacco use and body weight should be taken into consideration and corrected whenever possible. Similarly, the clinician must be aware of any chronic medical conditions that could be affected by this type of procedure or by pregnancy itself. One should also investigate for a patient or family history of clotting disorders.

Evaluation of the patient's ovarian reserve is mandatory for COH, because this assessment helps to anticipate excessive and/or untoward ovarian responses, and it provides guidance for selection of the starting gonadotropin dose. The two cornerstone indices of ovarian reserve are the AFC and plasma AMH. These measures usually vary in the same direction, but there is not yet a true consensus of normal ranges for these parameters. That said, an excessive response to stimulation should be anticipated when the total AFC is more than 24 follicles and/or the AMH level is above 6 ng/ml. Conversely, an insufficient response is likely when the total AFC is less than six follicles and/or the AMH level is lower than 1.0 ng/ml. It should be noted that while the AMH level correlates to some extent with the size of the recruited follicular cohort, it cannot predict oocyte quality or the chances for a successful pregnancy [3].

Several algorithms with multifactorial calculations have been proposed to establish the proper starting dose for each patient, but these typically approach only a probabilistic level [4]. Nevertheless the initial dose, which will be maintained for the first 5–6 stimulation days, is highly important for a harvest of 6–15 mature oocytes, the optimal number for achieving a live birth [5]. An insufficient starting dose will recruit a low follicle number that will not be corrected by further increases of posology; an excessive dose will provoke growth of too many follicles and a decrease of subsequent dosing may become very difficult to manage.

12.2.2 GnRH Analogues

Gonadotropin releasing hormone (GnRH, gonadorelin) is a decapeptide secreted in a pulsatile manner by hypothalamic neurons located primarily in the preoptic nucleus that project to the median eminence for secretion into portal vessels. Arcuate neurons project dopaminergic fibers that modulate GnRH release and suppress prolactin release. Upon transport via hypothalamic-pituitary portal vessels, GnRH binds to specific receptors on pituitary gonadotrophs. A pulsatile neuropeptide secretion signals a similar pattern of FSH and LH release that controls plasma gonadotropin levels, their circulating ratio, and also their relative bioactivity according to variations of their isoform composition.

The pituitary gonadotroph GnRH receptor is a G-coupled protein whose function follows the basic principle of desensitization. In order to exert a stimulating effect upon the gonadotropin secretion, the occupation of these receptors must be episodic, as is precisely the case with endogenous pulsatile GnRH secretion. When receptor occupation is maintained by continuous administration of GnRH or a high-affinity analogue, a tachyphylaxis occurs that terminates additional gonadotropin release. The intracellular subunits of the G-coupled GnRH receptor must reassemble in order to respond to another stimulus, but cannot do so while the peptide ligand remains bound to the outside binding domain. In order to be effective, GnRH administration must be pulsatile and this is accomplished through the use of a programmed pump. Continuous administration of GnRH is also possible if one wishes to terminate or down-regulate further gonadotropin release in order to reduce gonadal activity (Fig. 12.2).

Substitution of certain amino-acids of the GnRH decapeptide sequence creates analogues having different biological properties than the native hormone. However, the three first amino acids of the sequence are necessary for biological activity and the eight residue is essential for high affinity receptor binding (Fig. 12.3).

12.2.3 GnRH Agonists

A simple substitution of the l-alanine residue at position 6 or the l-glycine at position 10 with the respective dextrorotary enantiomer creates a potent agonist molecule because it gains an enhanced affinity for the GnRH receptor and the

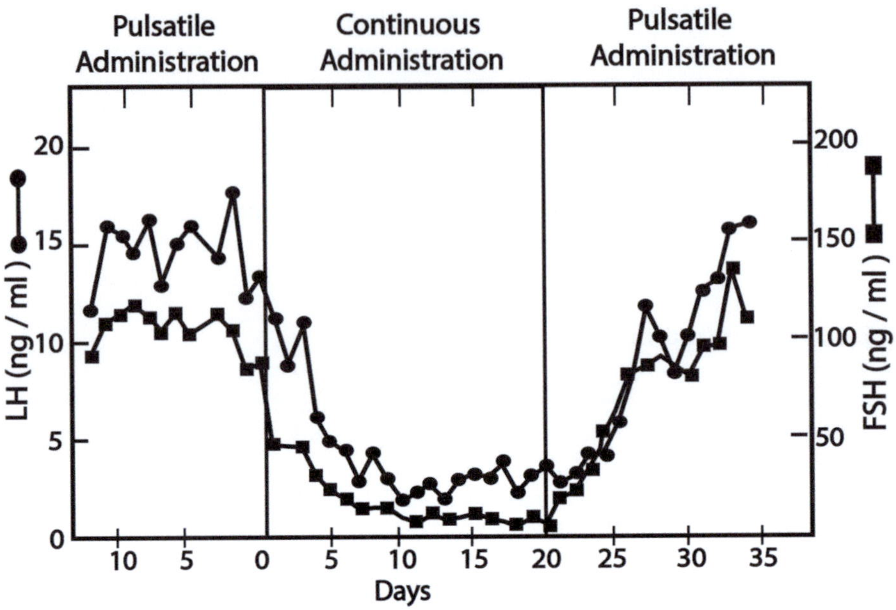

Fig. 12.2 The opposite effects of gonadorelin in accordance with its mode of administration

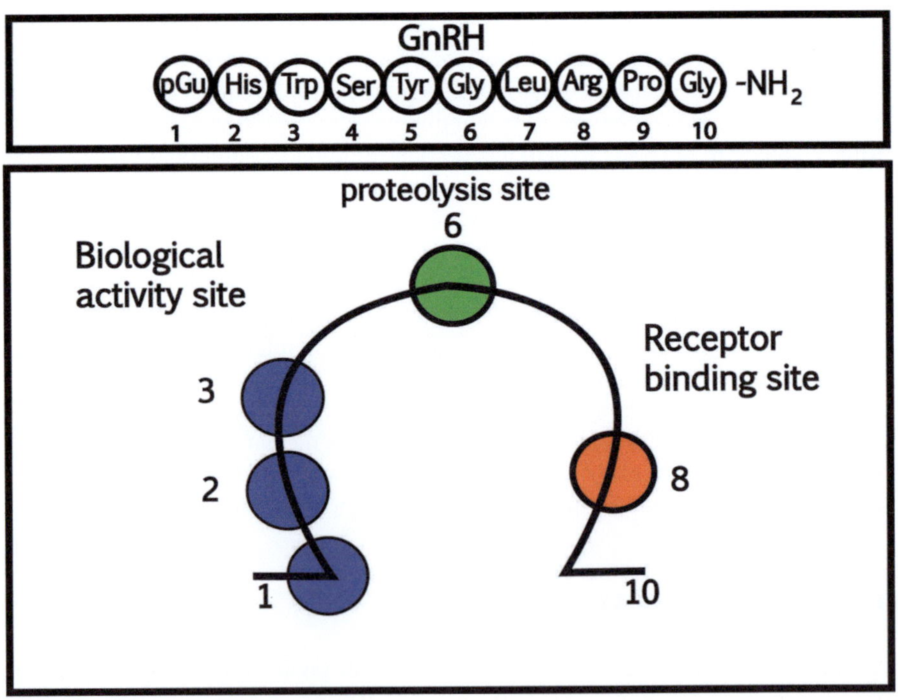

Fig. 12.3 Gonadorelin structure

Table 12.1 Structures of gonadotropin releasing hormone (GnRH, gonadorelin) and several analogs

		1	2	3	4	5	6	7	8	9	10	
	GONADORELIN	PYR	HIS	TRP	SER	TYR	GLY	LEU	ARG	PRO	GLY	– NH$_2$
AGONISTS	BUSERELIN	PYR	HIS	TRP	SER	TYR	D-Ser (BU)	LEU	ARG	PRO	ETHYLAMIDE	
	LEUPRORELIN	PYR	HIS	TRP	SER	TYR	D-LEU	LEU	ARG	PRO	ETHYLAMIDE	
	TRIPTORELIN	PYR	HIS	TRP	SER	TYR	D-TRP	LEU	ARG	PRO	GLY	– NH$_2$
	NAFARELIN	PYR	HIS	TRP	SER	TYR (NAPHTYL)	ALA	LEU	ARG	PRO	GLY	– NH$_2$
ANTAGONISTS	CETRORELIX	Ac D NaL	D Cpa	D PaL	SER	TYR	D Cit	LEU	ARG	PRO	D ALA	– NH$_2$
	GANIRELIX	Ac D NaL	D Cpa	D PaL	SER	TYR	D hARG	LEU	ARG	PRO	D ALA	– NH$_2$

structure resists degradation by plasma peptidases. These modified peptides retain a longer bioactive half-life and are effective at lower doses, which explains the contradictory effects of long acting agonists on gonadotropin secretion. An initial potent stimulation of gonadotropin release (the "flare up" effect) is quickly followed by a secondary inhibition due to residual occupation of receptors by the agonist. Continuous administration of native GnRH also produces a refractory desensitization of gonadotrophs. Similarly, prolonged administration of these modified agonists, either daily (in nasal sprays or by subcutaneous administration) or as injected depot preparations, results in FSH-LH suppression and a concomitant anovulation and reduction of ovarian steroids. This property is being used to advantage in various estrogen-dependent clinical conditions, from precocious puberty to endometriosis to hormone-dependent malignancy (Table 12.1).

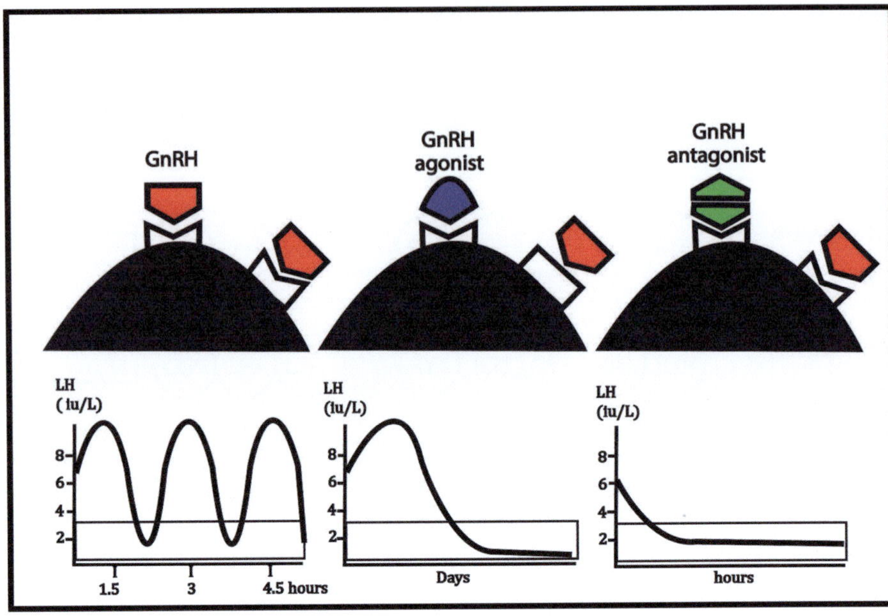

Fig. 12.4 Modes of action of GnRH agonists and antagonists

12.2.4 GnRH Antagonists

Substitution of the amino acids at positions 1, 2 and 3 of the decapeptide sequence results in loss of most of the biological activity, but the property of high-affinity receptor binding is preserved. This type of analogue acts as a GnRH antagonist: it binds to the receptor without an initial flare up effect while it prevents native GnRH from gaining receptor access (Fig. 12.4). A single administration has only a brief duration of action (about 24 h) and is reversed by use of GnRH itself or with one of the synthetic short lived agonists.

12.2.5 COH with GnRH Agonists

Use of GnRH agonists was introduced into multifollicular stimulation protocols for IVF purposes with the aim of preventing inappropriate LH surges. This controls the number of follicles reaching full maturity without risk that the more advanced ones would trigger a spontaneous ovulation. At present there are two protocols that differ in the timing of GnRH use:

The Short Protocol (Fig. 12.5). This utilizes only short-lived agonists, administered daily. Treatment starts on CD2 with the agonist alone for two days, then

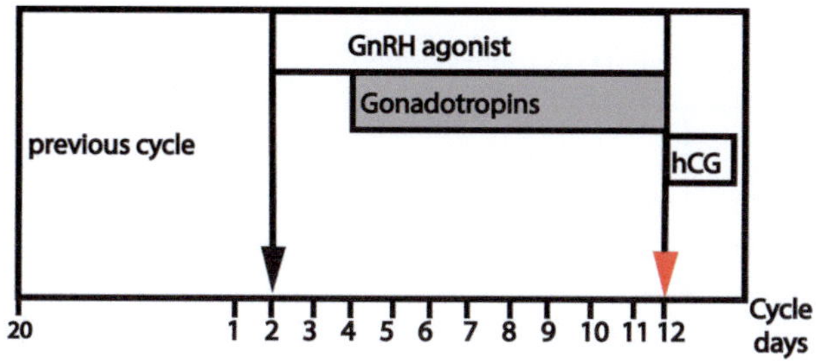

Fig. 12.5 Design of the short agonist protocol

gonadotropin injections are added from CD3 until ovulation. The two important effects of the agonist are at work:

- The initial stimulatory action provokes an FSH – LH surge that initiates follicular recruitment, roughly equivalent to a daily administration of 150 IU FSH.
- The subsequent pituitary tachyphylaxis permits exogenous ovarian stimulation through a full maturity of the follicular cohort but removes risk for a premature endogenous LH surge.

The first monitoring control should be done on CD6, the 5th stimulation day of four days GnRH agonist with two days gonadotropin administration added. Thereafter, assessments should be conducted at 2–3 day intervals according to the ovarian response (Table 12.2).

The Long Protocol (Fig. 12.6). This design introduces a new concept in ovarian stimulation, by exploiting even more the principle of pituitary desensitization. Stimulation itself is begun only after the ovaries have been put to rest by the prolonged withdrawal of endogenous gonadotropins following the agonist-induced shutdown of pituitary FSH and LH. The initial GnRH-induced flare up effect is not exploited in this protocol (Table 12.3). Ovarian activity ceases following daily administration of a short-lived GnRH agonist, or after a single injection of a long-acting GnRH agonist that lasts upwards of 1 month. In the latter case, gonadotropin administration should begin during the second half of the agonist effect, so that a possible embryo is not exposed to the GnRH analogue. Accordingly, gonadotropin administration begins 15–20 days after the agonist is administered, when ovarian shutdown has been established, and the injections continue under agonist control until the ovarian triggering.

Long-acting agonists may be administered on the first day of the cycle (a "follicular long-agonist" protocol), with the desensitization control and gonadotropin administration beginning on CD15. Alternatively, it may be started following ovulation (CD20) in the *previous* cycle (a "luteal long-agonist" protocol); in that case, desensitization control and gonadotropin administration should begin on CD 10 of the following cycle.

Table 12.2 Management of short agonist multifollicular protocol with a stimulation target of 6–14 follicles after 2 days of FSH (see StimXpert)

FD mm	< 9.9	10 - 12.9	13 - 14.9	15 - 16	>16
E2 pg/ml					
>2 500	S (4)	S (4)	2	1	S (4)
1 500 - 2 500	S (4)	3	2	1	hCG
750 - 1 500	S (4)	3	2	1	hCG
300-750	4	3	3	2	S (5) / hCG
100-300	4	3	3	2	S (3)
<100	4	3	2		S (3)

FSH
x 2 days

S	STOP
	+100%
	+50%
	100%
	-33%
	-50%
	0%

% of the starting dose

This table illustrates the types of decisions that should be made with various combinations of follicular response (FD mm, *top row*) and plasma estradiol (E_2 pg/ml, *left side column*)

Within each box, The *Circle Number* indicates the optimal number of days to continue stimulation, if triggering criteria have not yet been met after 2 days of stimulation. The *Circle Color* indicates the suggested percentage change for FSH dosing in relation to the previous (starting) dose. A *White Circle* with S indicates the cycle should be stopped or abandoned with no further stimulation. Boxes with HCG identify the follicle+estrogen criteria that permit ovulation triggering. Boxes with a number in parentheses refer to 1 of 3 footnotes listed below

Table 12.2 (continued)

When a patient is unable to come in for assessment after the indicated number of days, it remains possible to conduct the monitor one day earlier or later, possibly including a change of the FSH dose

The number of estradiol ranges has been purposely limited in order to simplify the table's construction, and should be considered as approximate when interpretations are made. In particular, when values are close to the indicated upper or lower value of E_2 within a range, the clinical decision should consider options indicated for the adjacent hormone level

Footnotes

1. Follicular growth that progresses faster than the rise of plasma estradiol levels may be related to an insufficient LH effect; in this case it is better to repeat the stimulation with an FSH preparation that includes LH
2. *Caution*: Risks for OHSS increase to the degree that plasma estradiol surpasses 2,500 pg/ml
3. A stimulation that progresses too rapidly (<7 days) may harm oocyte quality

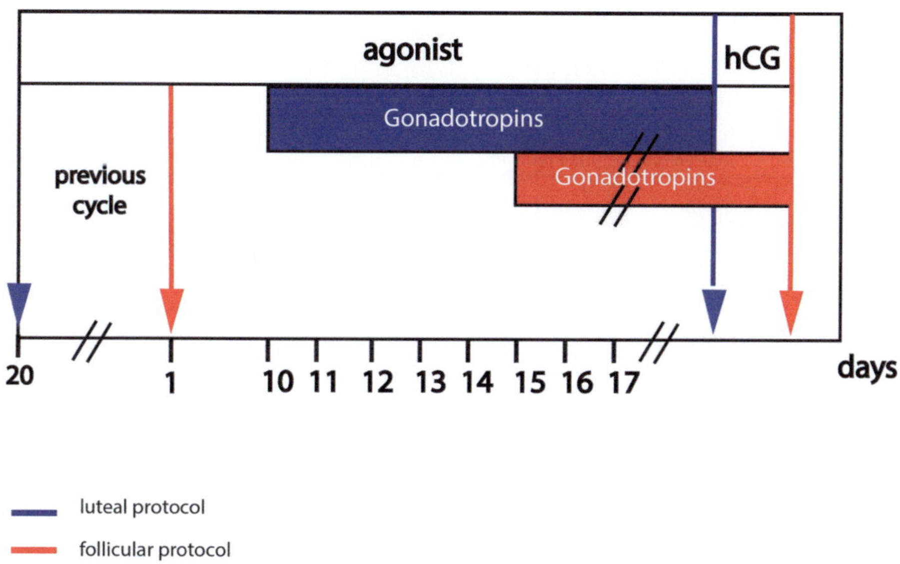

Fig. 12.6 Design of the long agonist protocol

Both protocols produce comparable results. Observations of functional ovarian cysts on the day of desensitization control are undoubtedly less frequent after the luteal administration protocol. On the other hand, the follicular administration protocol is the approach of choice in cases of irregular cycles, because administration on CD 20 of the previous cycle might intervene just before a late spontaneous ovulation and thus disorganize the following menses.

When complete ovarian rest is assured and gonadotropin administration is started, it is possible to reduce the daily dose of a short-lived agonist by half without risking a pituitary "escape" before triggering ovulation. Although this method was initially proposed for cases of poor ovarian response, it may be extended to all the patients.

Table 12.3 Management of long agonist multifollicular protocol with a stimulation target of 6–14 follicles after 5 days of FSH (see StimXpert)

FD mm	< 9.9	10 - 12.9	13 - 14.9	15 - 16	>16
E2 pg/ml					
>2 500	S (4)	S (4)	2 [white]	1 [white]	S (4)
1 500 - 2 500	S (4)	3 [blue]	2 [pink]	1 [pink]	hCG
750 - 1 500	3 [blue]	3 [pink]	2 [green]	1 [green]	hCG
300-750	4 [pink]	3 [pink]	3 [green]	2 [yellow]	S (5) / hCG
100-300	4 [green]	3 [green]	3 [yellow]	2 [red]	S (3)
<100	4 [red]	3 [red]	2 [red] / S (3)	S (3)	S (3)

FSH
x 5 days

S	STOP
[red]	+100%
[yellow]	+50%
[green]	100%
[pink]	-33%
[blue]	-50%
[white]	0%

% of the starting dose

This table illustrates the types of decisions that should be made with various combinations of follicular response (FD mm, *top row*) and plasma estradiol (E_2 pg/ml, *left side column*)

Table 12.3 (continued)

Within each box, The *Circle Number* indicates the optimal number of days to continue stimulation, if triggering criteria have not yet been met after 5 days of stimulation. The *Circle Color* indicates the suggested percentage change for FSH dosing in relation to the previous (starting) dose. A *White Circle* with S indicates the cycle should be stopped or abandoned with no further stimulation. Boxes with HCG identify the follicle+estrogen criteria that permit ovulation triggering. Boxes with a number in parentheses refer to 1 of 3 footnotes listed below

When a patient is unable to come in for assessment after the indicated number of days, it remains possible to conduct the monitor one day earlier or later, possibly including a change of the FSH dose

The number of estradiol ranges has been purposely limited in order to simplify the table's construction, and should be considered as approximate when interpretations are made. In particular, when values are close to the indicated upper or lower value of E_2 within a range, the clinical decision should consider options indicated for the adjacent hormone level

Footnotes

1. Follicular growth that progresses faster than the rise of plasma estradiol levels may be related to an insufficient LH effect; in this case it is better to repeat the stimulation with an FSH preparation that includes LH
2. *Caution*: Risks for OHSS increase to the degree that plasma estradiol surpasses 2,500 pg/ml
3. A stimulation that progresses too rapidly (<7 days) may harm oocyte quality

12.2.6 Choosing a GnRH Agonist

Long-acting depot agonists produce a more "depressed" pituitary gland than the ovarian rest obtained with daily injections of short-acting agonists. The latter usually leaves a basal level of gonadotropin secretion that daily agonist injections maintain at a minimal but not absent level. For this reason a greater total quantity of gonadotropins will be necessary to complete a stimulation cycle when long-acting formulations are used, because there is not even a low-level endogenous pituitary contribution.

None of the available GnRH agonists has been established as superior to any other insofar as pregnancy rates are concerned, and there are no reports of systematic prospective studies comparing one to another. On the other hand, patient responses may vary from one agonist to another, and a particular agonist may produce different results in different patients. This difference can be appreciated by examining the gonadotropin surge profile of the flare up effect, or by the comparative ability of various agonists to suppress FSH and LH in different patients. Thus one may consider changing to a different agonist in the same patient, from one COH to another.

Regardless of the ovarian appearance at ultrasound, pituitary suppression may be considered complete when plasma estradiol falls below 30 pg/ml. Ovarian ultrasound should reveal a number of follicles <6–8 mm accompanied by a thin linear uterine endometrium. Complete pituitary shutdown may not be reached by the time of the first examination. In these cases, continuation of the short agonist, or waiting several days longer after a depot long-acting agonist injection, may bring a more satisfactory ovarian rest.

It remains however possible that estradiol values will level off, or even increase while awaiting the moment to commence gonadotropin injections. In these cases, one may consider prolonging the cycle by immediate administration of another agonist and then repeating the assessment 15 days later. On rare occasions a paradoxical stimulatory effect of a depot agonist may occur, and a true ovarian hyperstimulation still remains possible. If ultrasound reveals numerous mature or pre-mature follicles in the presence of elevated serum estradiol levels, moving ahead with triggering the ovulation and retrieving oocytes seldom results in a successful pregnancy, and usually leads to a diminished chance for pregnancy in the patient [6]. In this situation it is preferable to cancel the cycle and prescribe 20 days of a potent oral progestin, whose anti-gonadotropic effect will return the ovaries to a resting state.

Once the desensitization is accomplished, ovarian stimulation may start, with an initial monitoring control made after 5–6 days of gonadotropin administration. Additional controls, basically intended to decide possible modifications of posology, are scheduled every two to three subsequent days. Two or three evaluations following the desensitization control will usually be necessary and sufficient.

12.2.7 Choosing a Gonadotropin Preparation

All of the available commercial preparations with an FSH effect produce essentially comparable pregnancy rates. The only question for clinicians is whether to add LH during the protocols, because use of GnRH agonists will suppress pituitary release of both gonadotropins. In fact, a large majority of patients maintain a residual, sufficient LH secretion, so administration of FSH alone should provide adequate ovarian stimulation. An essential minimal level for LH is estimated to be 1.2 IU/l. In theory, this identifies a need for serum LH monitoring, if a borderline endogenous LH secretion becomes insufficient for optimal follicular maturity. However, most LH assay kits are inadequately sensitive for accurate measures below 2 IU/l. Insufficient LH secretion may also be suspected when the follicular growth rate observed at ultrasound is rising faster than estradiol levels, but this kind of discrepancy may be very difficult to identify with a multifollicular cohort. The problem is manageable by changing the gonadotropin preparation and turning to an FSH+LH effect for successive cycles.

In summary, while the systematic supplementation of FSH with LH in agonist stimulation protocols does not yield better conception results overall, save for some older patients, the addition also has no recognized detrimental effect. There seems to be no overall difference in results obtained using pure FSH preparations versus those combining FSH and LH.

12.2.8 Choosing a Starting Dose

A starting dose of 150 IU seems best for the younger, normally-responsive patient. Higher doses are recommended for patients over 38 years of age, in those who are substantially overweight, or in those with a low ovarian reserve established by measures of AFC and/or AMH. Dosing level should also be diminished in the opposite situations.

Several algorithms have been proposed to calculate a priori the starting dose by means of several measured parameters, but it appears they only offer statistical data that may actually lead to erroneous assumptions for some patients [4, 5]. The number of possible starting doses being rather low, this dose may be calculated rather easily for most cases by listing the patient's age, her AFC or AMH level, and her BMI in a tabular fashion that increases or decreases the dose (Table 12.4).

12.2.9 Ovarian Responses to Monitor

Ovarian reactions to the gonadotropin administration may be evaluated according to two different approaches:

1. *Ovarian Sensitivity Index* (*OSI*), obtained by dividing the total number of gonadotropin units administered by the number of the oocytes harvested [7].
2. *Follicular Output RaTe* (*FORT*), obtained by multiplying the pre-ovulatory follicular count (PFC) on the triggering day by 100, then dividing by the AFC level on the day of desensitization control: $FORT = PFC \times 100/AFC$ [8]. Both of these parameters negatively correlate with the AMH level.

12.2.10 Criteria for Triggering

Among all the designed COH protocols, the long agonist protocol entails the greatest risk for ovarian hyperstimulation, if for no other reason that the process may be pursued without theoretical limits. There are likewise no generally acknowledged safety limits for the targeted number of follicles or the level of serum estradiol. Fertility teams tend to define their own limits in accordance with their own experiences and perceptions of various hazards. This question is further complicated in cases of COH because plasma estradiol levels, typically viewed as the best marker for OHSS risk, are poorly correlated with the follicular number due to the numerous (and safer) small follicles that still contribute to the estrogen pool. Estradiol level per follicle >14 mm diameter has been estimated to vary between 70 and 140 pg/ml [9], thus a maximum of 15 mature follicles together with an estradiol level ≤2,500 pg/ml would appear to be a reasonable upper limit. A higher estradiol level in the presence of numerous mature follicles would appear to be less hazardous than that same level in the presence of only a few mature follicles accompanied by a greater number of small and intermediate follicles.

In addition, the decision to trigger ovulation or to abandon the cycle is challenged by the unpredictable character of OHSS. On the one hand complications may not occur outside the safety limits, and on the other they may well happen within the safety range. The usual reason for pushing toward an OHSS is that clinicians are reluctant to cancel a cycle in uncertain circumstances when it can lead to further disillusionment for couples who have already invested so much.

Serum progesterone in excess of 1.5 ng/ml, on the morning of the scheduled triggering, may decrease the chances for pregnancy, undoubtedly because it disturbs the

Table 12.4 A simplified calculation schematic for the starting gonadotropin dose based on patient age, ovarian reserve (AFC or AMH level) and BMI

Parameter	-1	0	+1
AGE	< 33	34 - 38	> 39
AFC	>15	6 - 10	< 6
or AMH	> 6	2 - 6	< 2
BMI	< 17	29 - 18	> 30

	-3	-2	-1	0	+1	+2	+3
IU	75	75	100	150	225	300	300

Each of the three parameters can induce a 50 % increase or a 33 % reduction of the average starting dose (150 IU). The maximum range of changes remains between 75 IU (50 % reduction) and 300 IU (100 % increase)

implantation window, even as fertilization rates and embryonic development would appear unchanged. An elevated progesterone result should cause the cycle to be stopped, or alternatively the embryos should be frozen for implantation at a better moment, because the implantation ability of such embryos appears unaffected in another cycle [10]. Also, a rapid and short stimulation (less than 7 days) may result in suboptimal oocyte quality, and reduce the chances for success.

12.2.11 Comparing Short Versus Long Protocols

Both protocols were commenced as soon as the GnRH agonists appeared on the market, and their respective advantages and disadvantages became quickly recognized.

The short protocol, no matter the chosen strategy of use, has suffered from comparatively inferior rates of pregnancy. This deceptive advantage is explained in part by the protocol's tendency to develop smaller and less homogeneous follicular cohorts. Indeed, results are little improved over those observed with earlier protocols that did not include co-treatment with GnRH analogues.

The long protocol, however, has also been beset with some drawbacks, balanced by the critical benefit of pregnancy success to rates that were previously unknown. Among its major drawbacks is the need for a significantly larger quantity of administered gonadotropin per cycle. Higher FSH doses are necessary in order to reactivate the resting ovaries and also to drive the stimulation in the total absence of endogenous FSH. In addition, the prolonged pituitary-ovarian shutdown induces a form of menopausal syndrome of estrogen deprivation. Some patients may suffer hot flashes with sweats, headaches, and numerous other symptoms before the slowly developing stimulated follicles begin to replenish her estrogen. Many patients will recall this as the most difficult part of the entire IVF experience.

Nonetheless the advantages to the long protocol are also significant: the ovarian desensitization step of putting the ovaries to rest prior to beginning the stimulation induces a better, more homogeneous follicular cohort than with any of the other COH protocols in use. This poorly understood phenomenon results in greater numbers of high quality oocytes and embryos to select for fresh transfer or for freezing. Secondly, the monitoring process is made simpler because the ovaries have been basically disconnected from the pituitary and are responding only to the administered gonadotropins. A truly linear, almost monotonous stimulation is certainly the easiest to manage, save for the omnipresent risk for an OHSS. Thus, and perhaps most importantly, the rate of successful pregnancy was significantly higher than with any other COH protocol in use at that time, even as possible side effects, particularly on the endometrium, could not be ruled out. The long agonist protocol quickly became the gold standard for COH, and remains so for numerous IVF teams despite the evolution of other approaches following the appearance of GnRH antagonists.

12.2.12 COH with GnRH Antagonists

The availability of GnRH antagonists has permitted another approach for prevention of premature LH surges during the multifollicular simulation. This has also led to a more flexible protocol management because of the crucial differences in agonist-versus-antagonist effects on the pituitary gland.

First of all, an antagonist produces no initial stimulation of FSH-LH, as gonadotropin secretion ceases immediately. The effect can be reversed by an agonist within hours, whereas even a single administration of a short agonist is followed by a pituitary tachyphylaxis that persists for several days. Antagonists do not result in pituitary desensitization, even following a prolonged administration, and a normal pituitary response can be restored quickly by administration of gonadorelin or a synthetic congener. Antagonist protocols are of the short type, with gonadotropin administration starting as soon as the first days of the menstrual cycle.

12.2.13 Pre-treatment

The stimulation cycle may be prepared with a combination oral contraceptive during the cycle prior to stimulation, in order to prevent an inter-cycle rise of endogenous FSH. An alternate strategy is for the patient to take 4 mg oral micronized 17-β estradiol beginning on day 20 of the cycle prior to the planned stimulation. This has no recognized effect on the pregnancy rates, but it helps for the programming of oocyte retrieval. For example, one can begin gonadotropin administration on Wednesday through Friday of a week and thereby avoid ovarian punctures and laboratory work over the weekends [11].

12.2.14 Starting the Antagonist Administration

Gonadotropin stimulation can begin as soon as CD 2–3, or one to two days after discontinuation of the oral hormone pre-treatment, using a fixed dose for the first five stimulation days, until the first programmed monitoring control. At this point, two different antagonist protocols are possible depending upon the chosen moment of antagonist introduction.

1. *The "fixed" antagonist protocol*: Daily antagonist administration commences on the sixth stimulation day, no matter the prevailing follicular diameters and estradiol level, and is continued together with the gonadotropin injections until the triggering day (Fig. 12.7). Starting the antagonist as soon as the first day of the cycle, followed by gonadotropin administration starting on CD 2, has also been proposed with the aim of removing any residual endogenous LH effect on the recruited follicles, and this may be the preferred approach for hyperresponsive or PCOS patients [12]. Starting both antagonist and FSH administration on CD2 yields the same results.

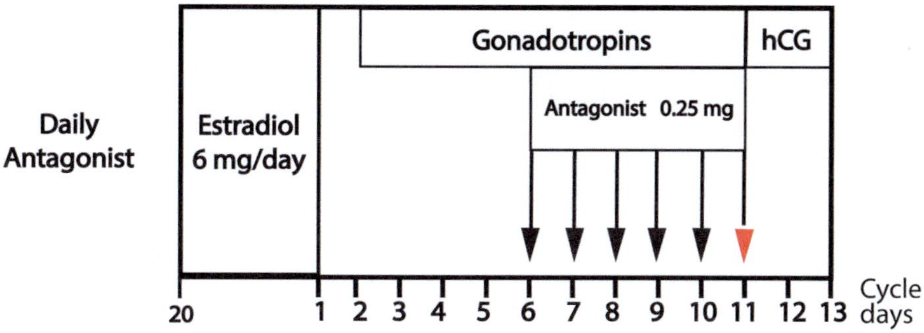

Fig. 12.7 Design of the fixed antagonist protocol

2. The "flexible" antagonist protocol: Antagonist administration is withheld until ultrasound and or hormonal criteria are reached. For example, one might begin when the leading follicle reaches 13–14 mm in diameter and/or plasma estradiol level exceeds 800 pg/ml (Table 12.5), on any CD.

Both protocols yield comparable results in terms of pregnancy rates: the fixed protocol usually results in more antagonist injections, but still remains as easy to manage as a short agonist stimulation. On the other hand, the flexible antagonist protocol usually requires fewer injections but needs more experience to conduct successfully, particularly to avoid starting the antagonist too late [13].

At present one can choose from two short lived antagonists for daily administration of 0.25 mg. A third preparation (cetrorelix 3 mg) designed for depot use and a 3-day duration effect is no longer available.

12.2.15 Revisiting Other Protocols with Antagonists

Suppression of LH surges without pituitary desensitization by using GnRH antagonists has led to improved management of some earlier developed protocols:

- The clomiphene-HMG/FSH protocol retains a main advantage of simplicity and a reduction of gonadotropin consumption. Criteria for introducing the GnRH antagonist remain the same, e.g., at the time of the initial monitoring control on CD9 [14].
- The natural cycle protocol tampers with the principal follicle only after it has been spontaneously recruited and selected. Concomitant daily administration of FSH and LH, usually as 150 IU HMG, plus a GnRH antagonist, can begin as soon as the follicular diameter reaches 14 mm. This helps sustain the selected follicle growth during the few days necessary to achieve optimal maturity, but without running the risk of a premature gonadotropin surge [15].

Table 12.5 Management of antagonist multifollicular protocol with a stimulation target of 5–10 follicles after 5 days of FSH (see StimXpert)

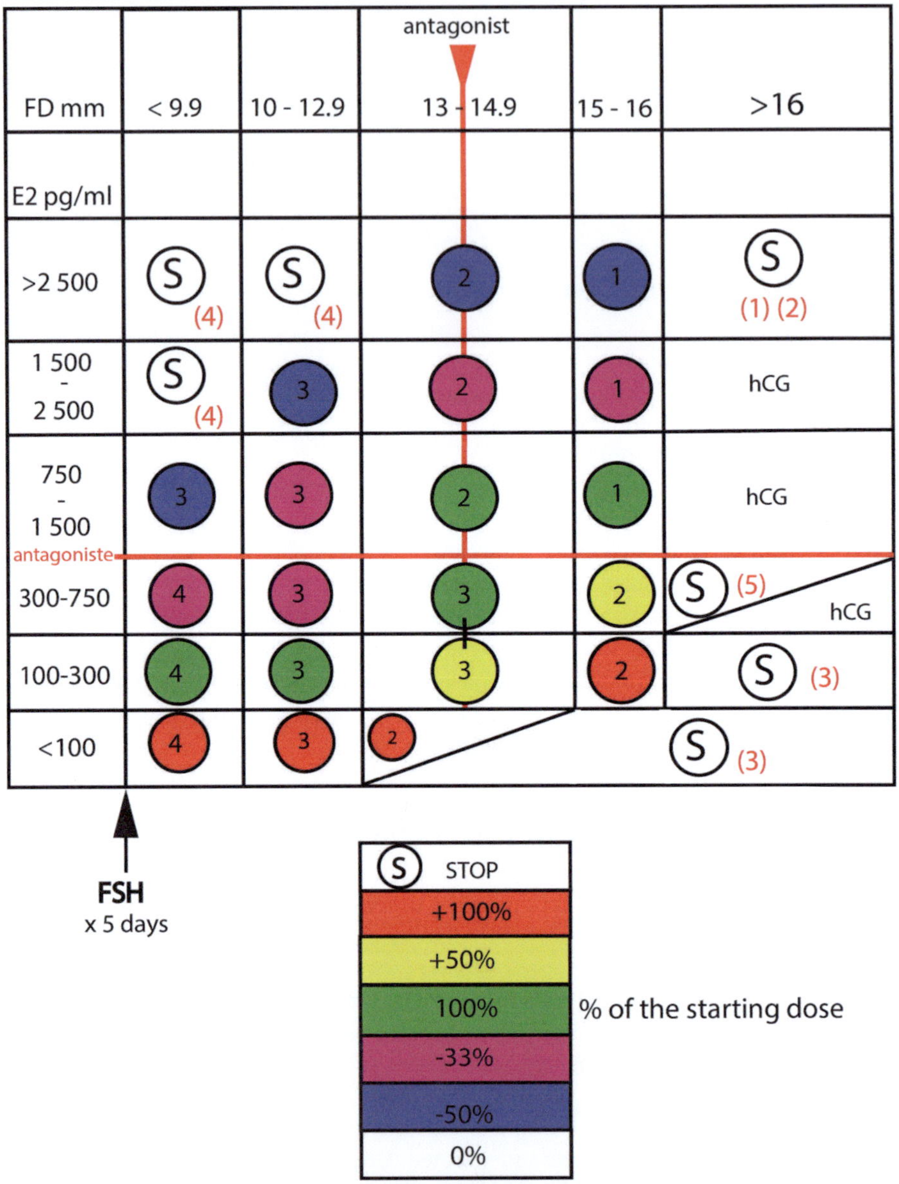

This table illustrates the types of decisions that should be made with various combinations of follicular response (FD mm, *top row*) and plasma estradiol (E_2 pg/ml, *left side column*)
Within each box, The *Circle Number* indicates the optimal number of days to continue stimulation, if triggering criteria have not yet been met after 5 days of stimulation. The *Circle Color* indicates the suggested percentage change for FSH dosing in relation to the previous (starting) dose. A *White Circle* with S indicates the cycle should be stopped or abandoned with no further stimulation. Boxes with HCG identify the follicle+estrogen criteria that permit ovulation triggering. Boxes with a number in parentheses refer to 1 of 4 footnotes listed below

Table 12.5 (continued)

When a patient is unable to come in for assessment after the indicated number of days, it remains possible to conduct the monitor one day earlier or later, possibly including a change of the FSH dose
The number of estradiol ranges has been purposely limited in order to simplify the table's construction, and should be considered as approximate when interpretations are made. In particular, when values are close to the indicated upper or lower value of E_2 within a range, the clinical decision should consider options indicated for the adjacent hormone level
Footnotes

1. Follicular growth that progresses faster than the rise of plasma estradiol levels may be related to an insufficient LH effect; in this case it is better to repeat the stimulation with an FSH preparation that includes LH
2. *Caution*: Risks for OHSS increase to the degree that plasma estradiol surpasses 800 pg/ml
3. A stimulation that progresses too rapidly may harm oocyte quality
4. Triggering with a short-acting agonist diminishes but does not completely eliminate risk of primary ovarian hyperstimulation syndrome

12.2.16 Recommendations for Management of the Stimulation (Table 12.5)

12.2.16.1 Selecting the Gonadotropin: Antagonist Combination

No particular combination of the various gonadotropin preparations and the two available antagonists has ever been established as superior. On the other hand, one combination may work best in certain patients, and for this reason it is best to consider changing the combination from one stimulation cycle to the next in the same patient.

12.2.16.2 Starting Doses?

In theory, initial FSH dosing should be set lower than those used in the long agonist protocols designed to "awaken" a resting ovary. In current practice, however, the same 150 IU starting dose seems best for all young normal responders. Dosing may need to be adjusted with respect to the patient's age, ovarian reserve, and BMI.

12.2.16.3 Schedule for Monitoring

An initial assessment should be done on the day of the first gonadotropin administration, to examine for a functional cyst, or an abnormally high progesterone level. A second ultrasound and hormonal sampling should be done on the sixth stimulation day, followed by additional assessments at two-to-three day intervals. Three or four evaluations should suffice. Although LH measures are not useful in the long agonist protocol, they become mandatory in this situation because of the risk for a pituitary "escape." While a single, isolated rise of LH (remaining under 10 IU/l) may still be effectively managed by administration of a GnRH antagonist, and not impact continuation of the cycle, a higher LH increment followed by a progesterone rise, no matter the reason, should cause the cycle to be stopped.

In addition, a rising progesterone level (>1.5 ng/ml) on the morning of the planned triggering, even in the absence of an LH surge, signals a possible ovulation escape, and could result in failure to harvest an oocyte during follicular puncture. In this situation one may choose to cancel the cycle or to continue with ovum retrieval and, if oocytes are harvested, to freeze all embryos for a later transfer. This avoids fresh transfers with an endometrium that is too mature.

12.2.16.4 Criteria for Triggering Ovulation

Criteria for triggering are the same as with the long agonist protocol, and are designed to yield a good follicular cohort (8–15 mature follicles) without risking an OHSS. Using a GnRH antagonist is very advantageous in this instance because the antagonism can be quickly reversed by administration of a short-acting agonist. This action results in an adequate final maturation of the follicles with resumption of meiosis, the only step of the ovulatory process that is still required when conducting IVF: follicular puncture replaces follicular rupture and luteal gland secretion is systematically supported by administration of progesterone. Subcutaneous injection of 0.2 mg triptorelin in place of hCG brings a substantial reduction of risk for early hyperstimulation, and does not appear to hamper oocyte harvest and quality. For these reasons, oocyte donor protocols consistently favor this agonist/antagonist approach.

However, triggering ovulation with an agonist in an antagonist protocol does have several drawbacks:

- Follicular puncture may fail to retrieve an oocyte despite careful follicular rinsing, if serum progesterone is < 3.5 mg/ml on the following morning [16].
- It may not prevent a late ovarian hyperstimulation, in the presence of an implanted embryo.
- It can be followed by a defective luteal phase and a dramatic decrease of implantation rate [17]. Progesterone administration alone or in association with micronized estradiol may not be sufficient, and co-administration of a small dose of hCG (750–1,500 IU) on the evening following follicular puncture will be necessary to rescue chances for pregnancy. Of course, the administration of hCG also restores a certain risk for early OHSS [18].

On the other hand, triggering ovulation with a GnRH agonist in an antagonist protocol provides better management of some hyperstimulation risks:

- *If "reasonable" risk of hyperstimulation*: trigger ovulation with hCG and complete the transfer.
- *If "high" risk*: trigger with a short-acting GnRH agonist, administer 750–1,500 IU hCG on the day of oocyte retrieval, and transfer. In questionable cases, hCG administration may be delayed as late as the 5th–6th day after ovum retrieval; this permits an assessment for early hyperstimulation before deciding on going ahead with the transfer.
- *If "highly critical" risk*: trigger ovulation with a short-acting agonist, do not support the luteal phase, refrain from completing the embryo transfer in the present cycle and freeze them for a later transfer. This policy does presume that the fertility center or clinic has satisfactory pregnancy rates with frozen embryos. Otherwise this situation could end with diminished chances of success for the patient.

Effective execution of these different strategies, which are becoming widely accepted among the IVF community, should result in a significant reduction, and possibly a total elimination, of OHSS secondary to COH, and to create at last a "hyperstimulation-free clinic."

12.2.17 The Unique Situation Regarding Corifollitropin Alpha

Corifollitropin is a "long acting" FSH preparation with effects lasting up to seven days following a single injection. Thus it is possible to start a stimulation protocol with a single FSH administration, conduct an initial monitoring assessment on Day 8, and continue the protocol with another gonadotropin preparation if triggering criteria have not been met at the first assessment. Use of this product contrasts with other FSH preparations in several ways:

- At present, corifollitropin is indicated only for patients with a normal ovarian reserve as determined by the usual criteria. There are not enough data yet on the use of this preparation in either hypersensitive or poor responders.
- The initial dose is determined by the patient's weight and age rather than her BMI, and only two dose sizes are available: 100 IU for patients <60 kg and up to 36 years of age; and 150 IU for patients ≥60 kg whatever their age, or >50 kg when they are >36 years of age.
- At the present time, only the fixed-antagonist protocol can use corifollitropin, because the initial monitoring control does not occur until the eight day following stimulation; at this moment, a gonadotropin surge may have already begun in some patients, so the GnRH antagonist needs to be introduced as soon as the sixth day following beginning of stimulation.

Depending upon the ultrasound and hormonal parameters observed on the eight day, the protocol proceeds from there in the same manner as would a fixed antagonist protocol conducted with any other FSH preparation.

12.2.18 Long Agonist and Antagonist Protocols

After an initial tumultuous period that included many enthusiastic reports following the introduction of this new stimulation tool, GnRH antagonist protocols began to disappoint many clinicians who were conducting controlled hyperstimulation procedures. Pregnancy rates calculated by oocyte retrieval or embryo transfer seemed significantly inferior to those of the long agonist protocol. Furthermore, antagonist management strategies seemed to bring more new questions (e.g., indications, product choice, preferred FSH preparation, and triggering criteria) to clinicians who were typically accustomed to the linear, almost monotonous process of long agonist protocols that usually produced more satisfaction than concerns [19]. It took the perseverance of a few groups dedicated to sustaining the antagonist protocols to begin convincing clinicians who were understandably reluctant to adopt changes that could threaten their pregnancy rates. Indeed, as with any new methodology, a certain learning curve is necessary to begin recognizing that an antagonist protocol can be managed with success in the same way as other multifollicular stimulation treatments [20]. At present, the two types of COH with GnRH analogues are recognized as offering rather the same chance for pregnancy, and it is now easy enough to evaluate their respective advantages and drawbacks [21].

The long agonist protocol has two main advantages: (1) a better, more homogeneous follicular cohort that results in a higher oocyte yield, (2) a simple management design that works well even with some approximations. The protocol also has significant drawbacks: (1) a longer duration of treatment that includes 10–15 days of agonist preparation prior to stimulation, (2) the agonist may induce an unpleasant period of estrogen withdrawal, (3) there is always a risk for OHSS that can prove difficult to manage, because an agonist triggering is not possible with this protocol.

The antagonist protocol includes many of the reverse characteristics. The main disadvantages are: (1) a smaller, less homogeneous follicular cohort that should still be sufficient to provide cumulative pregnancy rates comparable to those of the long agonist protocol, perhaps due to better oocyte quality, (2) the monitoring is less forgiving of management inaccuracies, insofar as the flexible protocol is concerned. Among the advantages are: (1) a shorter treatment duration with lower total doses of gonadotropins, (2) a better patient tolerance for the stimulation, due to the shorter treatment period and the absence of estrogen deprivation symptoms, and also with fewer injections when corifollitropin alpha is used, and (3) an easier management of risks for early ovarian hyperstimulation, principally because of the possibility of turning to a GnRH agonist in order to trigger ovulation. Increased use of the antagonist protocol has resulted in a better definition and refinement of the concept of the mild stimulation [22, 23].

12.2.19 Which COH Protocol Is Best?

This question remains difficult to answer directly, because it is generally acknowledged that all types of agonist and antagonist protocols yield comparable pregnancy rates when correctly managed. Some patients will become pregnant with almost any stimulation protocol while others will need a more customized approach. It is important to keep in mind that the patient should not be subject to the specifics of a protocol; rather, the protocol must submit to the specific aspects of each patient. Treatments should be adjusted according to the specific context, and other considerations:

- Each clinician should draw on his/her own experiences and greatest familiarity with the various protocols.
- For each patient, a particular FSH preparation should be chosen to match precisely a given GnRH analogue. This critical match may be difficult to foresee.
- For each IVF cycle to remain true to its objectives. Continuing progress in embryo technology permits the number of transferred embryos to be reduced, which of course lowers the risk of multiple pregnancies. The increasing use of the single embryo transfer strategy, with the same rate of successful pregnancy, makes it pointless, not to mention hazardous, to harvest a large number of oocytes, save for special situations like oocyte donation or fertility preservation.

For all these reasons, it seems less useful to search for the most ideal protocol in general, and more important to choose the best infertility work-up. Rather than repeatedly using the same FSH preparations with the same GnRH analogue, and with the same protocol for several IVF attempts, it seems preferable to follow a diversified strategy that encompasses the best chance to match a protocol correctly with each patient's problems and characteristics.

The Antagonist Protocol. Except for certain situations, co-treatment with a GnRH antagonist is perhaps the best stimulation approach for the first one or two attempts leading to in vitro fertilization:

- Most all patients who "implant well" will become pregnant no matter the stimulation protocol, and large follicular cohorts are not even needed.
- The antagonist protocol is a "kinder, gentler" stimulation that leaves fewer bad memories than does the long agonist treatment. This point is far from insignificant because too many patients with a good prognosis abandon their IVF program along with their hopes for pregnancy because of fear or the reality of uncomfortable stimulation procedures.
- The antagonist protocol is more applicable to all patient ages and levels of ovarian reserve. In patients with a lower follicular count, the long agonist treatment results in a difficult and less productive ovarian awakening in spite of higher FSH doses.
- The sequence of an antagonist protocol plus an agonist for triggering is becoming widely used when a large oocyte harvest is sought without a fresh transfer, such as for oocyte donation or fertility preservation programs.

The Long Agonist Protocol may become a better choice after one or two unsuccessful antagonist attempts, as the potential beneficial and harmful effects of the different GnRH analogues on the endometrium and implantation remain largely unknown. This approach may also be chosen as a first line stimulation in two different situations: (1) In case of endometriosis: the preliminary phase of estrogen deprivation, which may be prolonged for several weeks or even months, can have a positive effect on the symptoms of endometriosis as well as on the protocol and the chance for pregnancy. (2) In case a larger follicular cohort is desired for a fresh transfer: this could be useful for prolonged in vitro culture for blastocysts, or when a limited quantity of spermatozoa has been obtained by testicular epididymal sperm extraction (TESE).

Regardless of the protocol used, if the first IVF attempt fails, it is quite reasonable to consider changing it for the next COH, even if it is acknowledged that the chances for success do not rest on the sole ovarian stimulation. One can change FSH preparation and/or GnRH analogue with respect to starting doses and treatment management of the previous cycle. On the other hand, one may choose to repeat the same protocol when a clinical pregnancy of any duration was achieved previously.

These sorts of strategies undoubtedly have an empirical nature, but would any other strategy be totally devoid of this? If all attempts at IVF fail at last, the changes of protocol have the advantage of presenting the entire spectrum of available treatment options to the patient. In addition, those patients who explore the internet will be able to verify on their own the variety of possibilities that were undertaken.

Finally, clinicians should always be sensitive to the patient's comfort, and of ways to diminish untoward experiences by, for example, encouraging self-administered subcutaneous injections. Along the same line, there is little reason to impose a long agonist protocol of daily injections of triprorelin or buserelin, followed by two more daily injections (FSH and a GnRH agonist) when a single depot administration, or even nasal sprays of nafarelin or buserelin should yield the same results. Even when an IVF attempt fails, a COH achieves a certain bit of success when it does not leave the patient with unpleasant memories of this most difficult period of the IVF process, nor with anxiety about the next attempt. Keep in mind that giving up remains the primary cause of failure for patients undertaking IVF procedures.

12.3 In Case of Poor Ovarian Responses

In the COH process, the normal or average follicular response is generally agreed to be 6–14 ova. Fewer than six follicles is a weak response, 14–18 ova is a high response, and more than 18 is excessive. For an initial IVF attempt, a poor ovarian response (POR) is usually agreed to be three follicles or less. At a consensus conference that was recently convened in Bologna, Italy, a POR was defined when two of the following occur [24]:

- The patient is age 40 or older, or has additional risk factors for ovarian damage
- A POR (≤3 oocytes) observed in a previous COH with a long agonist protocol
- A poor ovarian reserve as measured by AFC (<5–6 follicles) and/or the AMH level (<0.5–1.0 ng/ml)

Together, these criteria include the circumstances by which a POR is discovered, either a priori, from the patient's age, history of ovarian damage, or abnormal ovarian reserve parameters; or a posteriori, following a deceptive COH. Nevertheless, these criteria can harbor surprises: while an expected POR may not occur, an inadequate response may remain fortuitous or be secondary to an erroneous starting dose of FSH.

Poor responses to ovarian stimulation typically share two characteristics: the occurrence rate increases with the patient's age and POR significantly diminishes the patient's chances for pregnancy. When making this diagnosis, it is very important to distinguish patients who should persevere in the process from those who will not and should turn instead to oocyte donation. Both are indeed heterogeneous populations but with different prognoses, which seems better for patients that have already conceived at least once. Quality of oocytes is not always correlated with quantity. Thus patients who fail to grow more than three oocytes during a stimulation trial can be divided into two categories [25]:

- Those with impaired oocyte quality because of age, or because of ovarian insufficiency from various causes at a younger age. These patients typically present with shorter menstrual cycles and higher FSH levels. Outlook for continued attempts at IVF remains deceptive.
- Those with good oocyte quality who should be encouraged to continue with IVF, in order to make good use of the few remaining oocytes that are more likely to produce an implanting embryo.

A number of approaches have been proposed in an effort to increase oocyte number in patients who demonstrate a limited number of FSH-responsive follicles per cycle.

12.3.1 In Preparation for the Stimulation

- *Oral estrogen +/− progestin.* The patient takes oral contraceptives or a 4 mg dose of micronized estradiol daily prior to a short agonist or an antagonist protocol, from 10 days before menses until 1–3 days before beginning gonadotropin administration. This serves to counteract an inter-cycle rise of FSH.
- *Growth hormone injections*, to stimulate synthesis of hepatic IGF1, which in turn enhances the FSH effect on ovarian granulosa cells. Daily administration of 8–12 IU should begin either 10 days before menses or at the beginning of the FSH stimulation, and should be continued until the day of triggering [26].
- *Oral dehydroepiandrosterone* (*DHEA*), 75 mg daily, beginning 6–12 weeks before the IVF attempt, has been proposed to enhance ovarian response, and with a cumulative effect over time [27]. This weak androgen, of ovarian and adrenocortical origin, is a pro-hormone for the follicular steroidogenesis, notably for testosterone. However a mechanism of action remains largely hypothetical. It may increase IGF1 synthesis and/or production of an intra-ovarian hormonal environment similar to the micropolycystic ovary situation with attendant abnormal transition between primordial and primary follicles.
- *Oral letrozole*, an inhibitor of aromatase. This compound, which lacks intrinsic hormonal activity, can stimulate ovulation and has been tested for this indication [28].

12.3.2 The Stimulation Protocol

The *long agonist protocol*, using a GnRH agonist administered daily, poses a challenge for low-responding ovaries to gonadotropins. One might consider reducing the agonist dose by half, or even stopping it altogether as soon as the FSH stimulation begins.

The *long agonist depot protocol*, which induces an even more profound ovarian shutdown, is clearly not suitable for the POR patient.

The *short agonist protocol* may be modified by using only microdoses, e.g., 0.05–0.025 mg triptorelin, when the regular daily dose is 0.1 mg, This should prevent an LH surge while leaving a sufficient residual of pituitary gonadotropin secretion [29, 30].

Antagonist protocols are generally well suited for POR treatment situations because there is no preliminary ovarian desensitization. Sequential short agonist/antagonist microdoses have also been proposed [31].

The spontaneous (natural) cycle may also be considered as a last resort in order to harvest a single oocyte with hope that the quality will be optimal after minimal hormonal manipulations [32]. This approach may be enhanced by using clomiphene 100–150 mg daily for five days starting on CD2, with a goal of growing an extra follicle.

12.3.3 The FSH Preparation

Addition of LH is believed to improve the ovarian response in these patients, even as they may show no detectable LH deficit [33]. Extracted gonadotropin preparations appear more appropriate when high doses are being administered, due to the "ceiling effect" of FSH.

12.3.4 The Starting Dose

Daily gonadotropin doses in excess of 300 IU are capable of inducing a better ovarian response in overweight patients whose POR had resulted from insufficient posology. In other patients, elevating the gonadotropin dose does not usually compensate for the lack of follicles sensitive to FSH [34]. Furthermore, increasing oocyte yield in these patients does not result in a higher pregnancy rate, perhaps because of the FSH ceiling effect. As a matter of fact, excessive FSH is counterproductive at the follicular level and actually may harm the oocyte quality. However it must be acknowledged that every clinic can report a few patients who achieved a successful pregnancy following daily administration of 450 IU or more FSH.

Conclusions

There is no single perfect multifollicular stimulation protocol for cases of POR related to the patient's age. No method appears superior to others, and furthermore none of them has been well validated [16]. Contradictory results appear in one publication or another and, inasmuch as the POR patients represent a heterogeneous group, the definition of POR itself remains a matter of debate. This deceptive situation confirms that the problem of the POR lies neither with the gonadotropin preparations nor with their administration protocols, but with conditions at the ovarian level itself. Nevertheless, it seems justified to continue with a few IVF attempts for these patients by testing some of these strategies in selected and motivated couples, after duly informing them of the empirical nature and uncertain outlook for these methods. The goal here is to pursue oocyte quality over oocyte quantity.

References

1. Steptoe PC, Edwards RG (1978) Birth after the reimplantation of a human embryo. Lancet 12:366
2. Emperaire JC, Ruffie A, Audebert AJM (1986) Fécondation *in vitro*: à la recherche du meilleur protocole de stimulation. Contracept Fertil Sexual 14:689–695
3. Loh S, Maheshwari A (2011) Anti-Mullerian hormone – is it a crystal ball for predicting ovarian aging ? Hum Reprod 36:2925–2932
4. Propovic-Todorovic B, Loft A et al (2003) A prospective, randomized clinical trial comparing an individual dose of recombinant FSH based on predictive factors versus a «standard» dose of 150 IU per day in «standard» patients undergoing IVF/ICSI treatment. Hum Reprod 18:2275–2282
5. Howles CM, Saunders H, Alam V, Engrand P (2006) Predictive factors and a corresponding treatment algorithm for controlled ovarian hyperstimulation in patients treated with recombinant human follicle stimulating hormone (follitropin alfa) during assisted reproductive technology (ART) procedures. An analysis of 1378 patients. Curr Med Res Opin 22:907–918
6. Pinto E, Pinelo S, Osorio M et al (2012) Outcomes from ovarian hyperstimulation following the sole administration of gonadotropin-releasing hormone agonist in the context of *in vitro* fertilization: report of two cases and review of the literature. Gynecol Endocrinol 28:545–548
7. Biasoni V, Patriarca A, Dalmasso P et al (2011) Ovarian sensitivity index is strongly correlated to circulating AMH and may be used to predict ovarian response to exogenous gonadotropins in IVF. Reprod Biol Endocrinol 9:112–116
8. Genro VK, Grynberg M, Scheffer JB et al (2011) Serum anti Müllerian hormone levels are negatively related to Follicular Output RaTe (FORT) in normo-cycling women undergoing controlled ovarian hyperstimulation. Hum Reprod 26:671–677
9. Loumaye E, Engrand P, Howles CM, O'Dean L (1997) Assessment of the role of serum luteinizing hormone and estradiol response to follicle stimulating hormone on *in vitro* fertilization treatment outcome. Fertil Steril 67:889–899
10. Huang R, Fang C, Xu S et al (2012) Premature progesterone rise negatively correlated with live birth rates in IVF cycles with GnRH agonist: an analysis of 2,566 cycles. Fertil Steril 98:664–670
11. Guivarc'h-Leveque A, Homer L, Arvis P et al (2011) Programming in vitro fertilization retrievals during working days after a gonadotropin-releasing hormone antagonist protocol with estrogen pretreatment: does the length of exposure to estradiol impact on controlled ovarian hyperstimulation outcomes? Fertil Steril 96:872–876
12. Montagut J, Nogueira D, Porcu G et al (2012) Administering GnRH antagonist from day 1 instead of day 7 in FIV/ICSI reduces OHSS: preliminary results of a randomized controlled trial on PCOS women. In: 27th annual meeting of the European Society of Human reproduction and embryology, Human Reprod 27 (Suppl 1) 2012
13. Emperaire JC (2004) Introduction of the antagonist: on a determined day or depending on follicular growth ? Gynecol Obstet Fertil 33(3S):39–41
14. Emperaire JC, Parneix I, Perraguin-Jayot S (2003) Revisiting the clomiphene-gonadotropin protocol in IVF with the use of a GnRH antagonist. Gynecol Obstet Fertil 31:917–931
15. Frydman R (2004) GnRH antagonists in natural cycle. J Gynecol Obstet Biol Reprod 33:46–49
16. Kummer NE, Feinn RS, Griffin DW et al (2013) Predicting successful induction of oocyte maturation after gonadotropin releasing hormone agonist (GnRH) trigger. Hum Reprod 145:56–61

17. Humaidan P, Ejdrup Bredkjaer H, Bungum L et al (2005) GnRH agonist (Buserelin) or HCG for ovulation induction in GnRH antagonist IVF/ICSI cycles : a prospective randomized study. Hum Reprod 20:1213–1220
18. Humaidan P, Ejdrup Bredkjaer H, Westergaard LG, Yding Andersen C (2010) 1500 IU human chorionic gonadotropin administered at oocyte retrieval rescues the luteal phase when gonadotropin-releasing hormone is used for ovulation induction: a prospective, randomized, controlled study. Fertil Steril 93:847–854
19. Tarlatzis BC, Fauser BC, Kolibianakis EM et al (2006) On behalf of the Brussels GnRH antagonist consensus workshop group. Hum Reprod Update 13:333–340
20. Emperaire JC, Parneix I (2007) Les antagonistes en FIV: Quelle place ? Quel monitorage ? Editions Frison-Roche, Paris
21. Olivennes F, Belaisch Allart J, Emperaire JC et al (2000) Prospective, randomized, controlled study of *in vitro* fertilization-embyro transfer with a single dose of luteinizing hormone-releasing hormone (LH-RH) antagonist (cetrorelix) or a depot formula of an LH-RH agonist (triptorelin). Fertil Steril 73:314–320
22. Emperaire JC (2006) Minimal ovarian stimulation: certainly less dangerous and probably as efficient. Gynecol Obstet Fertil 11:540–542
23. Fauser BC, Nargund G, Nyboe Andersen A (2010) Mild ovarian stimulation for IVF: 10 years later. Hum Reprod 25:2678–2684
24. Farraretti AP, LaMarca A, Fauser BC (2011) ESHRE consensus on the definition of "poor response" to ovarian stimulation for in vitro fertilization: the Bologna criteria. Hum Reprod 26:1616–1624
25. Oudendijk JF, Yarde F, Eijkemans MJC (2012) The poor responder in IVF: is the prognosis always poor ? A systematic review. Hum Reprod Update 18:1–11
26. De Ziegler D, Streuli I, Meldrum DR, Chapron C (2011) The value of growth hormone supplements in ART for poor ovarian responders. Fertil Steril 96:1069–1076
27. Wiser A, Gonen O, Ghetler Y et al (2010) Addition of dehydroepiandrosterone (DHEA) for poor responder patients before and during IVF treatment improves the pregnancy rate. A randomized prospective study. Hum Reprod 25:2496–2500
28. Lee VC, Chan CC, Ng EH et al (2011) Sequential use of letrozole and gonadotrophin in women with poor ovarian response. A randomized control trial. Reprod Biomed Online 23:380–388
29. Scott RT, Navot D (1994) Enhancement of ovarian responsiveness with microdoses of gonadotropin-releasing hormone during ovulation induction for *in vitro* fertilization. Fertil Steril 61:880–885
30. Park WI, Kim SS, Chung HR et al (2004) Early and late hormonal responses to the microdose gonadotropin-releasing hormone agonist in normal menstruating women. Fertil Steril 81:1067–1072
31. Ovieto R, Kruchkovich J, Rabinson J (2007) Ultrashort gonadotropin-releasing hormone agonist combined with flexible multidose gonadotropin-releasing hormone antagonist for poor responders in *in vitro* fertilization/embryo transfer programs. Fertil Steril 90:228–230
32. Reiftmann L, Dechaud H, Loup V et al (2007) Le cycle naturel en fécondation *in vitro* chez les mauvaises répondeuses. Gynecol Obstet Fertil 35:352–358
33. De Placido G, Alviggi C, Mollo A et al (2004) Effects of recombinant LH (rLH) supplementation during controlled ovarian hyperstimulation (COH) in normogonadotropic women with an initial inadequate response to recombinant FSH (rFSH) after pituitary downregulation. Clin Endocrinol 60:637–643
34. Berkkanoglu M, Ozgur K (2010) What is the maximal gonadotropin dosage used in microdose flare-up cycles in poor responders ? Fertil Steril 94:662–665

Conclusion

Stimulating ovulation with gonadotropins has proven through the years to be a very effective component of infertility management. Yet, to no surprise, success can also be accompanied by a number of significant hazards. For this reason it becomes essential to adopt some very precise rules of protocol that must be respected in order to ensure a harmonious as well as a safe stimulation. These rules include establishing an accurate diagnosis, recognizing appropriate goals, and adapting basic principles of ovulation induction to each patient's own situation.

One essential principle to remember is that no serious complication of the stimulation process will occur in the absence of hCG. Regardless of the protocol, intensity of the stimulation, or the nobility of objectives, hCG administration should be withheld when the situation develops an established risk, and carefully weighed even when the doubt arises. A trustworthy clinician must never turn the patient's problem of infertility into something worse.

Some patients will always be more difficult to stimulate than others, no matter the selected protocol and despite imaginative efforts undertaken to resolve the problem. Furthermore, ovulation stimulation remains far from an exact science: starting doses, dose adjustment, and intervals between monitoring controls will always require a practiced judgment that can reasonably be thought of as an art. In this regard, an estimation error or an unexpected downturn of conditions will always be possible at one moment or another. If an effective shift of strategy remains elusive, one has to be prepared to simply stop the treatment.

Everybody is of course conscious that a canceled cycle is an uncomfortable moment for all concerned, above all when it is not the first time. One must call upon a modest amount of courage to persuade the correct decision with the necessary, truthful explanations when a patient claims ownership of her own risks and responsibilities. A clinician must always retain sufficient self-control to disregard hopes for a magic touch or a guardian angel in order to avoid an unfortunate outcome.

Many patients are prematurely referred to assisted reproductive technology centers, only to be burdened with unnecessarily difficult procedures that would have been avoided with better management in their primary setting. Classic stimulation protocols are presently within reach of every gynecologist's practice. It would be advantageous for these clinicians to manage at least the initial steps of ART therapy for the patient who has already entrusted her care to his/her hands.

J.-C. Emperaire, *Ovulation Stimulation with Gonadotropins*,
DOI 10.1007/978-3-319-18654-2

MIX
Papier aus verantwortungsvollen Quellen
Paper from responsible sources
FSC® C105338

If you have any concerns about our products,
you can contact us on
ProductSafety@springernature.com

In case Publisher is established outside the EU,
the EU authorized representative is:
Springer Nature Customer Service Center GmbH
Europaplatz 3, 69115 Heidelberg, Germany

Printed by Libri Plureos GmbH
in Hamburg, Germany